Food Journal & Blood Sugar Log

I. S. Anderson

Food Journal & Blood Sugar Log

For more information regarding this publication, contact:
nahjpress@outlook.com

First Printing, 2015

Contents

Part One

- How to Use this Journal
- Sample Pages
- Counting Added Sugar

Part Two
- Starting Statistics and Goals
- Food and Blood Sugar Records

Part Three
- Weekly Progress Report and Graph
- Additional Graphs
- Nutrition Facts

How to Use this Journal

Starting Statistics and Goals: Define your diet/weight loss goals at the beginning of your journey and discuss how you plan to achieve them. Note that your **Food Journal & Blood Sugar Log** can be used for three months of dieting or to track shorter sessions.

Sleep: Begin each day by recording the number of hours you slept. A good night's sleep is one of the keys to good health and evidence suggests that those who get less than seven hours of sleep per night are more likely to gain weight.[12] Note that skimping on sleep, even a little, can affect your mood, energy, ability to handle stress, productivity, and mental sharpness.

Food/Beverage: Record the food and beverages you consume for the day, including the serving size, and the time you ate. Try to write this within 15 minutes of eating. Additional information can be provided in the title bar of each meal, such as your mood, who you had your meal with, and where. Note that you have the option of tracking one or more of the following food counts: calories, carbohydrates (carbs), added sugar, fiber, protein, and fat.

Vitamins/Supplements/Meds: Record any vitamins, supplements, or medications you take. Include the time you took them and the quantity.

Physical Activities: Record your physical activities for the day.

Nutrition Index: A nutrition index is provided at the back of the journal. Use the "Commonly Eaten Foods" page to build your own reference guide for the foods you eat on a regular basis.

Weekly Progress Report and Graphs: Use the *Weekly Progress Report* to update your statistics and to chart your progress over the next three months. Graphs are provided to track your weight and/or any other activities that you deem important.

---

[1] *Brondel L, Romer MA, Nougues PM, Touyarou P, Davenne D. Acute partial sleep deprivation increases food intake in healthy men. Am J Clin Nutr. 2010;91:1550–9.*

[2] *Patel SR, Malhotra A, White DP, et al. Association between reduced sleep and weight gain in women. Am J Epidemiol . 2006;164(10):947–954.*

Sample Pages

Day: 5   03 / 04 / 2015   Weight: 145
(Date)

Sleep (hrs): 1 2 3 4 5 6 7 8

	Calories	Carbs (g)	Added Sugar (g)	Fiber (g)	Protein (g)	Fat (g)
BREAKFAST						
2 cups oatmeal	286	51	0	7	10	
1 tbsp honey	64	17	16	0	0	
1 tbsp raisins	27	7	0	0	0	
1 oz almonds	172	5	0	3	6	
Time: 7:00 Totals:	549	80	16	10	16	
SNACK *feeling tired*						
1 medium apple	72	19	0	3	0	
1 cup coffee - black	2					
Time: 10:00 Totals:	74	19	0	3	0	
LUNCH *with Cheryl*						
2 cups chicken soup	193	12	0	1	11	
w/dumplings						
Time: 12:30 Totals:	193	12	0	1	11	
SNACK						
1 cup cashews	755	39	0	4	22	
1 can (12 oz) soda	114	49	47	0	0	
Time: 3:00 Totals:	869	88	47	4	22	
Page Totals:	1685	199	63	18	49	

VITAMINS/SUPPLEMENTS/MEDS.

7:00 Vit. C - 500 mg   12:30 Vit. D - 2000 IUs

Sample Pages (Cont'd)

Water: 1 2 3 4 5 6 7 8
(8 oz)

	Calories	Carbs (g)	Added Sugar (g)	Fiber (g)	Protein (g)	Fat (g)
DINNER *alone - very tired*						
Chicken leg 1/4, baked	180	0	0	0	25	
2 cups brown rice	244	44	0	3	5	
1 cup salad - avocado,						
tomato, lettuce, carrots						
no dressing	90	9	0	4	2	
8 oz iced tea, no sugar	2	1	0	0	0	
Time: 7:30 Totals:	516	54	0	7	32	
SNACK						
Time: Totals:						
Grand Totals:	2201	253	63	25	81	

PHYSICAL ACTIVITY

Activity	Duration	Intensity	Cal/Burn
Tennis with Jillian	1 hr.	High	
Walked	30 mins	Low	

BLOOD SUGAR LOG

	Before	After	Insulin
Breakfast	70	123	
Lunch	120	160	
Dinner	180	210	
Bedtime			

NOTES:
Was tired all day - didn't get enough sleep

Counting Added Sugar

What you should know:

- There are two types of sugar:
    o **Naturally occurring sugars** - these can be found in milk, fruits, and vegetables
    o **Added sugars** – sugars and syrups that are added to foods and beverages during processing

- 1 teaspoon of sugar = 4 grams

- 4 grams of sugar = 16 calories

- The average American consumes 22.2 teaspoons of added sugar per day or 355 calories.[3]

- The American Heart Health Association recommends that Americans reduce their sugar intake to no more than 100 calories per day for women and 150 calories per day for men.

- Soft drinks and other sweetened beverages are the primary source of added sugars in the American diet

- Food labels do not make the distinction between natural sugars and added sugars. Instead, the term *sugar* is used to refer to total sugars per serving.

- The following terms are used to describe added sugar:
    o Dextrose, fructose, honey, invert sugar, raw sugar, malt syrup, rice syrup, sucrose, xylose, molasses, corn sweetener, fruit juice, concentrate, high fructose corn syrup, brown sugar, glucose, lactose, maltose, sucrose, evaporated cane juice, agave nectar, cane crystals, cane sugar, crystalline fructose, barley malt, beet sugar, caramel

---

[3] *Dietary sugars intake and cardiovascular health: a scientific statement from the American Heart Association.*

Counting added sugar:

1. If the food is an unprocessed item (e.g. fruit or vegetable) there is no added sugar.

2. If the item is a prepared food, check the ingredients for one or more of the terms used to describe added sugar. Once you have identified one (or more), you now have proof that sugar has been added.

3. If the item contains natural sugars from milk, fruits, or vegetables, plus added sugar, then you will need to subtract the natural sugars.

4. Let's start counting:

   Apple, blueberry granola (1/4 cup)
   - **Ingredients**: Whole grain oats, <u>evaporated cane juice</u>, rice flour, mixed fruit concentrate, unsulfured dried apples, oat flour, natural blueberry flavor, tocopherols (vitamin E)
   - Source of natural sugars = no
   - Total carbohydrates = 33 g; Sugars = 12 g
   - Added sugars = 12 g

   Plain low fat yogurt (6 oz):
   - **Ingredients:** Cultured grade A reduced fat milk, pectin
   - Source of natural sugars = yes;
   - Total carbohydrate = 12 g; Sugars = 12 g
   - Added sugar = 0

   Low fat yogurt – coffee (6 oz):
   - **Ingredients**: Cultured grade A reduced fat milk, <u>sugar</u>, natural coffee flavor (including coffee extract), natural flavor, pectin
   - Source of natural sugars = yes
   - Total carbohydrates: 26 g; Sugars = 25 g
   - Added sugars: 13 g (plain yogurt has 12 g so, 25-12)

Food & Blood Sugar Records

Starting Statistics and Goals

Date: _____/_____/_____

		CURRENT	GOALS
BLOOD SUGAR			
Fasting	mg/dL	_____	_____
Before meals	mg/dL	_____	_____
After meals	mg/dL	_____	_____
EXERCISE			
Workout time	minutes per day	_____	_____
Other exercises	minutes per day	_____	_____
MEASUREMENTS			
Blood pressure	reading	_____	_____
Weight	pounds/stones	_____	_____
Upper arms	inches/cm	_____	_____
Chest	inches/cm	_____	_____
Waist	inches/cm	_____	_____
Hips	inches/cm	_____	_____
Thighs	inches/cm	_____	_____
_____	inches/cm	_____	_____
_____	inches/cm	_____	_____
FOOD & BEVERAGE			
Calories	per day	_____	_____
Fat	grams per day	_____	_____
Protein	grams per day	_____	_____
Carbohydrates	grams per day	_____	_____
_____	grams per day	_____	_____
_____	grams per day	_____	_____

To achieve these goals, I will:

_____
_____
_____
_____
_____

Starting Statistics and Goals

Date: _____ / _____ / _____

BLOOD SUGAR		CURRENT	GOALS
Fasting	mg/dL	_____	_____
Before meals	mg/dL	_____	_____
After meals	mg/dL	_____	_____

EXERCISE

Workout time	minutes per day	_____	_____
Other exercises	minutes per day	_____	_____

MEASUREMENTS

Blood pressure	reading	_____	_____
Weight	pounds/stones	_____	_____
Upper arms	inches/cm	_____	_____
Chest	inches/cm	_____	_____
Waist	inches/cm	_____	_____
Hips	inches/cm	_____	_____
Thighs	inches/cm	_____	_____
_____	inches/cm	_____	_____
_____	inches/cm	_____	_____

FOOD & BEVERAGE

Calories	per day	_____	_____
Fat	grams per day	_____	_____
Protein	grams per day	_____	_____
Carbohydrates	grams per day	_____	_____
_____	grams per day	_____	_____
_____	grams per day	_____	_____

To achieve these goals, I will: _____
_____
_____
_____
_____
_____

Day: [ ]   2 / 13 / 23   **Weight:** 239
                      (Date)

Sleep (hrs): 1 2 3 4 5 (6) 7 8

	Calories	Carbs (g)	Added Sugar (g)	Fiber (g)	Protein (g)	Fat (g)
BREAKFAST 6 AM						
2 buttered toast						
Time: Totals:						
SNACK 10 AM						
3 cheese slices						
Time: Totals:						
LUNCH						
Time: Totals:						
SNACK						
Time: Totals:						
Page Totals:						

VITAMINS/SUPPLEMENTS/MEDS.

Water: 1 2 3 4 5 6 7 8
(8 oz)

	Calories	Carbs (g)	Added Sugar (g)	Fiber (g)	Protein (g)	Fat (g)
DINNER						
Time: Totals:						
SNACK						
Time: Totals:						
Grand Totals:						

PHYSICAL ACTIVITY

Activity	Duration	Intensity	Cal/Burn

BLOOD SUGAR LOG

	Before	After	Insulin
Breakfast	123		14 H
Lunch	119		
Dinner			
Bedtime			

NOTES:

Day: [ ]   ___/___/___   Weight: [ ]
                    (Date)

Sleep (hrs): 1 2 3 4 5 6 7 8

	Calories	Carbs (g)	Added Sugar (g)	Fiber (g)	Protein (g)	Fat (g)
BREAKFAST						
Time: Totals:						
SNACK						
Time: Totals:						
LUNCH						
Time: Totals:						
SNACK						
Time: Totals:						
Page Totals:						

VITAMINS/SUPPLEMENTS/MEDS.

Water: 1 2 3 4 5 6 7 8
(8 oz)

	Calories	Carbs (g)	Added Sugar (g)	Fiber (g)	Protein (g)	Fat (g)
DINNER						
Time: Totals:						
SNACK						
Time: Totals:						
Grand Totals:						

PHYSICAL ACTIVITY

Activity	Duration	Intensity	Cal/Burn

BLOOD SUGAR LOG

	Before	After	Insulin
Breakfast			
Lunch			
Dinner			
Bedtime			

NOTES:

Day: [ ] ____/____/____ Weight: [ ]
(Date)

Sleep (hrs): 1 2 3 4 5 6 7 8

	Calories	Carbs (g)	Added Sugar (g)	Fiber (g)	Protein (g)	Fat (g)
BREAKFAST						
Time: Totals:						
SNACK						
Time: Totals:						
LUNCH						
Time: Totals:						
SNACK						
Time: Totals:						
Page Totals:						

VITAMINS/SUPPLEMENTS/MEDS.

Water: 1 2 3 4 5 6 7 8
(8 oz)

	Calories	Carbs (g)	Added Sugar (g)	Fiber (g)	Protein (g)	Fat (g)	
DINNER							
Time: Totals:							
SNACK							
Time: Totals:							
Grand Totals:							

PHYSICAL ACTIVITY

Activity	Duration	Intensity	Cal/Burn

BLOOD SUGAR LOG

	Before	After	Insulin
Breakfast			
Lunch			
Dinner			
Bedtime			

NOTES:

_____
_____
_____
_____
_____

Day: [ ] ____/____/____ **Weight:** [ ]
(Date)

Sleep (hrs): 1 2 3 4 5 6 7 8

	Calories	Carbs (g)	Added Sugar (g)	Fiber (g)	Protein (g)	Fat (g)
BREAKFAST						
Time: Totals:						
SNACK						
Time: Totals:						
LUNCH						
Time: Totals:						
SNACK						
Time: Totals:						
Page Totals:						

VITAMINS/SUPPLEMENTS/MEDS.

Water: 1 2 3 4 5 6 7 8
(8 oz)

DINNER	Calories	Carbs (g)	Added Sugar (g)	Fiber (g)	Protein (g)	Fat (g)
Time: Totals:						
SNACK						
Time: Totals:						
Grand Totals:						

PHYSICAL ACTIVITY

Activity	Duration	Intensity	Cal/Burn

BLOOD SUGAR LOG

	Before	After	Insulin
Breakfast			
Lunch			
Dinner			
Bedtime			

NOTES:

Day: [ ]   ____/____/____   Weight: [ ]

(Date)

Sleep (hrs): 1 2 3 4 5 6 7 8

	Calories	Carbs (g)	Added Sugar (g)	Fiber (g)	Protein (g)	Fat (g)
BREAKFAST						
Time: Totals:						
SNACK						
Time: Totals:						
LUNCH						
Time: Totals:						
SNACK						
Time: Totals:						
Page Totals:						

VITAMINS/SUPPLEMENTS/MEDS.

[ ]

Water: 1 2 3 4 5 6 7 8
(8 oz)

	Calories	Carbs (g)	Added Sugar (g)	Fiber (g)	Protein (g)	Fat (g)
DINNER						
Time: Totals:						
SNACK						
Time: Totals:						
Grand Totals:						

PHYSICAL ACTIVITY

Activity	Duration	Intensity	Cal/Burn

BLOOD SUGAR LOG

	Before	After	Insulin
Breakfast			
Lunch			
Dinner			
Bedtime			

NOTES:

Day: [ ] ____/____/____
(Date) **Weight:** [ ]

Sleep (hrs): 1 2 3 4 5 6 7 8

	Calories	Carbs (g)	Added Sugar (g)	Fiber (g)	Protein (g)	Fat (g)
BREAKFAST						
Time: Totals:						
SNACK						
Time: Totals:						
LUNCH						
Time: Totals:						
SNACK						
Time: Totals:						
Page Totals:						

VITAMINS/SUPPLEMENTS/MEDS.

[ ]

Water: 1 2 3 4 5 6 7 8
(8 oz)

	Calories	Carbs (g)	Added Sugar (g)	Fiber (g)	Protein (g)	Fat (g)
DINNER						
Time: Totals:						
SNACK						
Time: Totals:						
Grand Totals:						

PHYSICAL ACTIVITY

Activity	Duration	Intensity	Cal/Burn

BLOOD SUGAR LOG

	Before	After	Insulin
Breakfast			
Lunch			
Dinner			
Bedtime			

NOTES:
_____
_____
_____
_____
_____

Day: [ ]   ____/____/____   Weight: [ ]
                     (Date)

Sleep (hrs): 1 2 3 4 5 6 7 8

	Calories	Carbs (g)	Added Sugar (g)	Fiber (g)	Protein (g)	Fat (g)
BREAKFAST						
Time: Totals:						
SNACK						
Time: Totals:						
LUNCH						
Time: Totals:						
SNACK						
Time: Totals:						
Page Totals:						

VITAMINS/SUPPLEMENTS/MEDS.

[ ]

Water: 1 2 3 4 5 6 7 8
(8 oz)

	Calories	Carbs (g)	Added Sugar (g)	Fiber (g)	Protein (g)	Fat (g)
DINNER						
Time: Totals:						
SNACK						
Time: Totals:						
Grand Totals:						

PHYSICAL ACTIVITY

Activity	Duration	Intensity	Cal/Burn

BLOOD SUGAR LOG

	Before	After	Insulin
Breakfast			
Lunch			
Dinner			
Bedtime			

NOTES:

Day: [ ]   ____/____/____   **Weight:** [ ]

(Date)

Sleep (hrs): 1 2 3 4 5 6 7 8

	Calories	Carbs (g)	Added Sugar (g)	Fiber (g)	Protein (g)	Fat (g)
BREAKFAST						
Time: Totals:						
SNACK						
Time: Totals:						
LUNCH						
Time: Totals:						
SNACK						
Time: Totals:						
Page Totals:						

VITAMINS/SUPPLEMENTS/MEDS.

Water: 1 2 3 4 5 6 7 8
(8 oz)

	Calories	Carbs (g)	Added Sugar (g)	Fiber (g)	Protein (g)	Fat (g)
DINNER						
Time: Totals:						
SNACK						
Time: Totals:						
Grand Totals:						

PHYSICAL ACTIVITY

Activity	Duration	Intensity	Cal/Burn

BLOOD SUGAR LOG

	Before	After	Insulin
Breakfast			
Lunch			
Dinner			
Bedtime			

NOTES:

Day: ☐   ___/___/___   **Weight:** ☐
(Date)

Sleep (hrs): 1 2 3 4 5 6 7 8

	Calories	Carbs (g)	Added Sugar (g)	Fiber (g)	Protein (g)	Fat (g)
BREAKFAST						
Time: Totals:						
SNACK						
Time: Totals:						
LUNCH						
Time: Totals:						
SNACK						
Time: Totals:						
Page Totals:						

VITAMINS/SUPPLEMENTS/MEDS.

Water: 1 2 3 4 5 6 7 8
(8 oz)

	Calories	Carbs (g)	Added Sugar (g)	Fiber (g)	Protein (g)	Fat (g)	
DINNER							
Time: Totals:							
SNACK							
Time: Totals:							
Grand Totals:							

PHYSICAL ACTIVITY

Activity	Duration	Intensity	Cal/Burn

BLOOD SUGAR LOG

	Before	After	Insulin
Breakfast			
Lunch			
Dinner			
Bedtime			

NOTES:

Day: ☐　　　＿＿＿／＿＿＿／＿＿＿　　**Weight:** ☐
　　　　　　　　　　　(Date)

Sleep (hrs): 1 2 3 4 5 6 7 8

	Calories	Carbs (g)	Added Sugar (g)	Fiber (g)	Protein (g)	Fat (g)
BREAKFAST						
Time:　　　Totals:						
SNACK						
Time:　　　Totals:						
LUNCH						
Time:　　　Totals:						
SNACK						
Time:　　　Totals:						
Page Totals:						

VITAMINS/SUPPLEMENTS/MEDS.

Water: 1 2 3 4 5 6 7 8
(8 oz)

	Calories	Carbs (g)	Added Sugar (g)	Fiber (g)	Protein (g)	Fat (g)
DINNER						
Time: Totals:						
SNACK						
Time: Totals:						
Grand Totals:						

PHYSICAL ACTIVITY

Activity	Duration	Intensity	Cal/Burn

BLOOD SUGAR LOG

	Before	After	Insulin
Breakfast			
Lunch			
Dinner			
Bedtime			

NOTES:

Day: [ ]   ____/ ____/ ____   Weight: [   ]
                        (Date)

Sleep (hrs): 1 2 3 4 5 6 7 8

	Calories	Carbs (g)	Added Sugar (g)	Fiber (g)	Protein (g)	Fat (g)	
BREAKFAST							
Time: Totals:							
SNACK							
Time: Totals:							
LUNCH							
Time: Totals:							
SNACK							
Time: Totals:							
Page Totals:							

VITAMINS/SUPPLEMENTS/MEDS.

[   ]

Water: 1 2 3 4 5 6 7 8
(8 oz)

	Calories	Carbs (g)	Added Sugar (g)	Fiber (g)	Protein (g)	Fat (g)
DINNER						
Time: Totals:						
SNACK						
Time: Totals:						
Grand Totals:						

PHYSICAL ACTIVITY

Activity	Duration	Intensity	Cal/Burn

BLOOD SUGAR LOG

	Before	After	Insulin
Breakfast			
Lunch			
Dinner			
Bedtime			

NOTES:

Day: ⬚   ____/____/____   **Weight:** ⬚
(Date)

Sleep (hrs): 1 2 3 4 5 6 7 8

	Calories	Carbs (g)	Added Sugar (g)	Fiber (g)	Protein (g)	Fat (g)
BREAKFAST						
Time: Totals:						
SNACK						
Time: Totals:						
LUNCH						
Time: Totals:						
SNACK						
Time: Totals:						
Page Totals:						

VITAMINS/SUPPLEMENTS/MEDS.

Water: 1 2 3 4 5 6 7 8
(8 oz)

	Calories	Carbs (g)	Added Sugar (g)	Fiber (g)	Protein (g)	Fat (g)	
DINNER							
Time: Totals:							
SNACK							
Time: Totals:							
Grand Totals:							

PHYSICAL ACTIVITY

Activity	Duration	Intensity	Cal/Burn

BLOOD SUGAR LOG

	Before	After	Insulin
Breakfast			
Lunch			
Dinner			
Bedtime			

NOTES:

Day: ☐   ____ / ____ / _____   Weight: ☐

(Date)

Sleep (hrs): 1 2 3 4 5 6 7 8

	Calories	Carbs (g)	Added Sugar (g)	Fiber (g)	Protein (g)	Fat (g)
BREAKFAST						
Time: Totals:						
SNACK						
Time: Totals:						
LUNCH						
Time: Totals:						
SNACK						
Time: Totals:						
Page Totals:						

VITAMINS/SUPPLEMENTS/MEDS.

Water: 1 2 3 4 5 6 7 8
(8 oz)

	Calories	Carbs (g)	Added Sugar (g)	Fiber (g)	Protein (g)	Fat (g)
DINNER						
Time: Totals:						
SNACK						
Time: Totals:						
Grand Totals:						

PHYSICAL ACTIVITY

Activity	Duration	Intensity	Cal/Burn

BLOOD SUGAR LOG

	Before	After	Insulin
Breakfast			
Lunch			
Dinner			
Bedtime			

NOTES:

Day: [ ]   ___/___/___   **Weight:** [ ]
(Date)

Sleep (hrs): 1 2 3 4 5 6 7 8

	Calories	Carbs (g)	Added Sugar (g)	Fiber (g)	Protein (g)	Fat (g)
BREAKFAST						
Time: Totals:						
SNACK						
Time: Totals:						
LUNCH						
Time: Totals:						
SNACK						
Time: Totals:						
Page Totals:						

VITAMINS/SUPPLEMENTS/MEDS.

[ ]

Water: 1 2 3 4 5 6 7 8
(8 oz)

	Calories	Carbs (g)	Added Sugar (g)	Fiber (g)	Protein (g)	Fat (g)
DINNER						
Time: Totals:						
SNACK						
Time: Totals:						
Grand Totals:						

PHYSICAL ACTIVITY

Activity	Duration	Intensity	Cal/Burn

BLOOD SUGAR LOG

	Before	After	Insulin
Breakfast			
Lunch			
Dinner			
Bedtime			

NOTES:

Day: [ ]   ____/____/____   Weight: [ ]
                      (Date)

Sleep (hrs): 1 2 3 4 5 6 7 8

	Calories	Carbs (g)	Added Sugar (g)	Fiber (g)	Protein (g)	Fat (g)	
BREAKFAST							
Time: Totals:							
SNACK							
Time: Totals:							
LUNCH							
Time: Totals:							
SNACK							
Time: Totals:							
Page Totals:							

VITAMINS/SUPPLEMENTS/MEDS.

```



```

Water: 1 2 3 4 5 6 7 8
(8 oz)

	Calories	Carbs (g)	Added Sugar (g)	Fiber (g)	Protein (g)	Fat (g)
DINNER						
Time: Totals:						
SNACK						
Time: Totals:						
Grand Totals:						

PHYSICAL ACTIVITY

Activity	Duration	Intensity	Cal/Burn

BLOOD SUGAR LOG

	Before	After	Insulin
Breakfast			
Lunch			
Dinner			
Bedtime			

NOTES:

Day: ☐   ____ / ____ / ____   **Weight:** ☐
(Date)

Sleep (hrs): 1 2 3 4 5 6 7 8

	Calories	Carbs (g)	Added Sugar (g)	Fiber (g)	Protein (g)	Fat (g)
BREAKFAST						
Time: Totals:						
SNACK						
Time: Totals:						
LUNCH						
Time: Totals:						
SNACK						
Time: Totals:						
Page Totals:						

VITAMINS/SUPPLEMENTS/MEDS.

Water: 1 2 3 4 5 6 7 8
(8 oz)

	Calories	Carbs (g)	Added Sugar (g)	Fiber (g)	Protein (g)	Fat (g)
DINNER						
Time: Totals:						
SNACK						
Time: Totals:						
Grand Totals:						

PHYSICAL ACTIVITY

Activity	Duration	Intensity	Cal/Burn

BLOOD SUGAR LOG

	Before	After	Insulin
Breakfast			
Lunch			
Dinner			
Bedtime			

NOTES:

Day: ☐   ___/___/___   Weight: ☐

(Date)

Sleep (hrs): 1 2 3 4 5 6 7 8

	Calories	Carbs (g)	Added Sugar (g)	Fiber (g)	Protein (g)	Fat (g)
BREAKFAST						
Time: Totals:						
SNACK						
Time: Totals:						
LUNCH						
Time: Totals:						
SNACK						
Time: Totals:						
Page Totals:						

VITAMINS/SUPPLEMENTS/MEDS.

Water: 1 2 3 4 5 6 7 8
(8 oz)

	Calories	Carbs (g)	Added Sugar (g)	Fiber (g)	Protein (g)	Fat (g)
DINNER						
Time: Totals:						
SNACK						
Time: Totals:						
Grand Totals:						

PHYSICAL ACTIVITY

Activity	Duration	Intensity	Cal/Burn

BLOOD SUGAR LOG

	Before	After	Insulin
Breakfast			
Lunch			
Dinner			
Bedtime			

NOTES:

Day: [ ]   ____ / ____ / ____   **Weight:** [ ]
(Date)

Sleep (hrs): 1 2 3 4 5 6 7 8

	Calories	Carbs (g)	Added Sugar (g)	Fiber (g)	Protein (g)	Fat (g)	
BREAKFAST							
Time: Totals:							
SNACK							
Time: Totals:							
LUNCH							
Time: Totals:							
SNACK							
Time: Totals:							
Page Totals:							

VITAMINS/SUPPLEMENTS/MEDS.

Water: 1 2 3 4 5 6 7 8
(8 oz)

	Calories	Carbs (g)	Added Sugar (g)	Fiber (g)	Protein (g)	Fat (g)
DINNER						
Time: Totals:						
SNACK						
Time: Totals:						
Grand Totals:						

PHYSICAL ACTIVITY

Activity	Duration	Intensity	Cal/Burn

BLOOD SUGAR LOG

	Before	After	Insulin
Breakfast			
Lunch			
Dinner			
Bedtime			

NOTES:

Day: [ ] _____/_____/_____ Weight: [ ]
(Date)

Sleep (hrs): 1 2 3 4 5 6 7 8

	Calories	Carbs (g)	Added Sugar (g)	Fiber (g)	Protein (g)	Fat (g)
BREAKFAST						
Time: Totals:						
SNACK						
Time: Totals:						
LUNCH						
Time: Totals:						
SNACK						
Time: Totals:						
Page Totals:						

VITAMINS/SUPPLEMENTS/MEDS.

Water: 1 2 3 4 5 6 7 8
(8 oz)

DINNER	Calories	Carbs (g)	Added Sugar (g)	Fiber (g)	Protein (g)	Fat (g)
Time: Totals:						
SNACK						
Time: Totals:						
Grand Totals:						

PHYSICAL ACTIVITY

Activity	Duration	Intensity	Cal/Burn

BLOOD SUGAR LOG

	Before	After	Insulin
Breakfast			
Lunch			
Dinner			
Bedtime			

NOTES:

Day: ☐   ____ / ____ / ____   **Weight:** ☐
                    (Date)

Sleep (hrs): 1 2 3 4 5 6 7 8

	Calories	Carbs (g)	Added Sugar (g)	Fiber (g)	Protein (g)	Fat (g)
BREAKFAST						
Time: Totals:						
SNACK						
Time: Totals:						
LUNCH						
Time: Totals:						
SNACK						
Time: Totals:						
Page Totals:						

VITAMINS/SUPPLEMENTS/MEDS.

Water: 1 2 3 4 5 6 7 8
(8 oz)

	Calories	Carbs (g)	Added Sugar (g)	Fiber (g)	Protein (g)	Fat (g)
DINNER						
Time: Totals:						
SNACK						
Time: Totals:						
Grand Totals:						

PHYSICAL ACTIVITY

Activity	Duration	Intensity	Cal/Burn

BLOOD SUGAR LOG

	Before	After	Insulin
Breakfast			
Lunch			
Dinner			
Bedtime			

NOTES:

Day: ☐   ____/____/____   **Weight:** ☐
                    (Date)

Sleep (hrs): 1 2 3 4 5 6 7 8

	Calories	Carbs (g)	Added Sugar (g)	Fiber (g)	Protein (g)	Fat (g)
BREAKFAST						
Time: Totals:						
SNACK						
Time: Totals:						
LUNCH						
Time: Totals:						
SNACK						
Time: Totals:						
Page Totals:						

VITAMINS/SUPPLEMENTS/MEDS.

Water: 1 2 3 4 5 6 7 8
(8 oz)

	Calories	Carbs (g)	Added Sugar (g)	Fiber (g)	Protein (g)	Fat (g)
DINNER						
Time: Totals:						
SNACK						
Time: Totals:						
Grand Totals:						

PHYSICAL ACTIVITY

Activity	Duration	Intensity	Cal/Burn

BLOOD SUGAR LOG

	Before	After	Insulin
Breakfast			
Lunch			
Dinner			
Bedtime			

NOTES:

Day: [ ] ____/____/____ Weight: [ ]
(Date)

Sleep (hrs): 1 2 3 4 5 6 7 8

	Calories	Carbs (g)	Added Sugar (g)	Fiber (g)	Protein (g)	Fat (g)
BREAKFAST						
Time: Totals:						
SNACK						
Time: Totals:						
LUNCH						
Time: Totals:						
SNACK						
Time: Totals:						
Page Totals:						

VITAMINS/SUPPLEMENTS/MEDS.

Water: 1 2 3 4 5 6 7 8
(8 oz)

	Calories	Carbs (g)	Added Sugar (g)	Fiber (g)	Protein (g)	Fat (g)	
DINNER							
Time: Totals:							
SNACK							
Time: Totals:							
Grand Totals:							

PHYSICAL ACTIVITY

Activity	Duration	Intensity	Cal/Burn

BLOOD SUGAR LOG

	Before	After	Insulin
Breakfast			
Lunch			
Dinner			
Bedtime			

NOTES:

Day: [ ] ___/___/___   **Weight:** [ ]
(Date)

Sleep (hrs): 1 2 3 4 5 6 7 8

	Calories	Carbs (g)	Added Sugar (g)	Fiber (g)	Protein (g)	Fat (g)
BREAKFAST						
Time: Totals:						
SNACK						
Time: Totals:						
LUNCH						
Time: Totals:						
SNACK						
Time: Totals:						
Page Totals:						

VITAMINS/SUPPLEMENTS/MEDS.

[ ]

Water: 1 2 3 4 5 6 7 8
(8 oz)

	Calories	Carbs (g)	Added Sugar (g)	Fiber (g)	Protein (g)	Fat (g)
DINNER						
Time: Totals:						
SNACK						
Time: Totals:						
Grand Totals:						

PHYSICAL ACTIVITY

Activity	Duration	Intensity	Cal/Burn

BLOOD SUGAR LOG

	Before	After	Insulin
Breakfast			
Lunch			
Dinner			
Bedtime			

NOTES:

Day: ⬜   ___/___/___   Weight: ⬜
              (Date)

Sleep (hrs): 1 2 3 4 5 6 7 8

	Calories	Carbs (g)	Added Sugar (g)	Fiber (g)	Protein (g)	Fat (g)
BREAKFAST						
Time: Totals:						
SNACK						
Time: Totals:						
LUNCH						
Time: Totals:						
SNACK						
Time: Totals:						
Page Totals:						

VITAMINS/SUPPLEMENTS/MEDS.

Water: 1 2 3 4 5 6 7 8
(8 oz)

	Calories	Carbs (g)	Added Sugar (g)	Fiber (g)	Protein (g)	Fat (g)
DINNER						
Time: Totals:						
SNACK						
Time: Totals:						
Grand Totals:						

PHYSICAL ACTIVITY

Activity	Duration	Intensity	Cal/Burn

BLOOD SUGAR LOG

	Before	After	Insulin
Breakfast			
Lunch			
Dinner			
Bedtime			

NOTES:

Day: [ ]   _____/_____/_____   **Weight:** [ ]

(Date)

Sleep (hrs): 1 2 3 4 5 6 7 8

	Calories	Carbs (g)	Added Sugar (g)	Fiber (g)	Protein (g)	Fat (g)
BREAKFAST						
Time: Totals:						
SNACK						
Time: Totals:						
LUNCH						
Time: Totals:						
SNACK						
Time: Totals:						
Page Totals:						

VITAMINS/SUPPLEMENTS/MEDS.

Water: 1 2 3 4 5 6 7 8
(8 oz)

	Calories	Carbs (g)	Added Sugar (g)	Fiber (g)	Protein (g)	Fat (g)
DINNER						
Time: Totals:						
SNACK						
Time: Totals:						
Grand Totals:						

PHYSICAL ACTIVITY

Activity	Duration	Intensity	Cal/Burn

BLOOD SUGAR LOG

	Before	After	Insulin
Breakfast			
Lunch			
Dinner			
Bedtime			

NOTES:

Day: ☐   ____/ ____/ ____   **Weight:** ☐

(Date)

Sleep (hrs): 1 2 3 4 5 6 7 8

	Calories	Carbs (g)	Added Sugar (g)	Fiber (g)	Protein (g)	Fat (g)
BREAKFAST						
Time: Totals:						
SNACK						
Time: Totals:						
LUNCH						
Time: Totals:						
SNACK						
Time: Totals:						
Page Totals:						

VITAMINS/SUPPLEMENTS/MEDS.

Water: 1 2 3 4 5 6 7 8
(8 oz)

	Calories	Carbs (g)	Added Sugar (g)	Fiber (g)	Protein (g)	Fat (g)
DINNER						
Time: Totals:						
SNACK						
Time: Totals:						
Grand Totals:						

PHYSICAL ACTIVITY

Activity	Duration	Intensity	Cal/Burn

BLOOD SUGAR LOG

	Before	After	Insulin
Breakfast			
Lunch			
Dinner			
Bedtime			

NOTES:

Day: [ ]   ____/____/____   **Weight:** [ ]
                        (Date)

Sleep (hrs): 1 2 3 4 5 6 7 8

	Calories	Carbs (g)	Added Sugar (g)	Fiber (g)	Protein (g)	Fat (g)
BREAKFAST						
Time: Totals:						
SNACK						
Time: Totals:						
LUNCH						
Time: Totals:						
SNACK						
Time: Totals:						
Page Totals:						

VITAMINS/SUPPLEMENTS/MEDS.

Water: 1 2 3 4 5 6 7 8
(8 oz)

	Calories	Carbs (g)	Added Sugar (g)	Fiber (g)	Protein (g)	Fat (g)
DINNER						
Time: Totals:						
SNACK						
Time: Totals:						
Grand Totals:						

PHYSICAL ACTIVITY

Activity	Duration	Intensity	Cal/Burn

BLOOD SUGAR LOG

	Before	After	Insulin
Breakfast			
Lunch			
Dinner			
Bedtime			

NOTES:

Day: [ ]   ____/____/____   Weight: [ ]
                     (Date)

Sleep (hrs): 1 2 3 4 5 6 7 8

	Calories	Carbs (g)	Added Sugar (g)	Fiber (g)	Protein (g)	Fat (g)
BREAKFAST						
Time: Totals:						
SNACK						
Time: Totals:						
LUNCH						
Time: Totals:						
SNACK						
Time: Totals:						
Page Totals:						

VITAMINS/SUPPLEMENTS/MEDS.

[ ]

Water: 1 2 3 4 5 6 7 8
(8 oz)

	Calories	Carbs (g)	Added Sugar (g)	Fiber (g)	Protein (g)	Fat (g)
DINNER						
Time: Totals:						
SNACK						
Time: Totals:						
Grand Totals:						

PHYSICAL ACTIVITY

Activity	Duration	Intensity	Cal/Burn

BLOOD SUGAR LOG

	Before	After	Insulin
Breakfast			
Lunch			
Dinner			
Bedtime			

NOTES:

Day: [ ]   ___/___/___   Weight: [ ]
                    (Date)

Sleep (hrs): 1 2 3 4 5 6 7 8

	Calories	Carbs (g)	Added Sugar (g)	Fiber (g)	Protein (g)	Fat (g)
BREAKFAST						
Time: Totals:						
SNACK						
Time: Totals:						
LUNCH						
Time: Totals:						
SNACK						
Time: Totals:						
Page Totals:						

VITAMINS/SUPPLEMENTS/MEDS.

Water: 1 2 3 4 5 6 7 8
(8 oz)

DINNER	Calories	Carbs (g)	Added Sugar (g)	Fiber (g)	Protein (g)	Fat (g)
Time: Totals:						
SNACK						
Time: Totals:						
Grand Totals:						

PHYSICAL ACTIVITY

Activity	Duration	Intensity	Cal/Burn

BLOOD SUGAR LOG

	Before	After	Insulin
Breakfast			
Lunch			
Dinner			
Bedtime			

NOTES:

Day: ☐   _____/_____/_____   **Weight:** ☐
                       (Date)

Sleep (hrs): 1 2 3 4 5 6 7 8

	Calories	Carbs (g)	Added Sugar (g)	Fiber (g)	Protein (g)	Fat (g)
BREAKFAST						
Time: Totals:						
SNACK						
Time: Totals:						
LUNCH						
Time: Totals:						
SNACK						
Time: Totals:						
Page Totals:						

VITAMINS/SUPPLEMENTS/MEDS.

Water: 1 2 3 4 5 6 7 8
(8 oz)

	Calories	Carbs (g)	Added Sugar (g)	Fiber (g)	Protein (g)	Fat (g)
DINNER						
Time: Totals:						
SNACK						
Time: Totals:						
Grand Totals:						

PHYSICAL ACTIVITY

Activity	Duration	Intensity	Cal/Burn

BLOOD SUGAR LOG

	Before	After	Insulin
Breakfast			
Lunch			
Dinner			
Bedtime			

NOTES:

Day: [ ]   ____/____/____   Weight: [ ]

(Date)

Sleep (hrs): 1 2 3 4 5 6 7 8

	Calories	Carbs (g)	Added Sugar (g)	Fiber (g)	Protein (g)	Fat (g)
BREAKFAST						
Time: Totals:						
SNACK						
Time: Totals:						
LUNCH						
Time: Totals:						
SNACK						
Time: Totals:						
Page Totals:						

VITAMINS/SUPPLEMENTS/MEDS.

Water: 1 2 3 4 5 6 7 8
(8 oz)

	Calories	Carbs (g)	Added Sugar (g)	Fiber (g)	Protein (g)	Fat (g)
DINNER						
Time: Totals:						
SNACK						
Time: Totals:						
Grand Totals:						

PHYSICAL ACTIVITY

Activity	Duration	Intensity	Cal/Burn

BLOOD SUGAR LOG

	Before	After	Insulin
Breakfast			
Lunch			
Dinner			
Bedtime			

NOTES:

Day: [ ]   ____/____/____   Weight: [ ]
                    (Date)

Sleep (hrs): 1 2 3 4 5 6 7 8

	Calories	Carbs (g)	Added Sugar (g)	Fiber (g)	Protein (g)	Fat (g)
BREAKFAST						
Time: Totals:						
SNACK						
Time: Totals:						
LUNCH						
Time: Totals:						
SNACK						
Time: Totals:						
Page Totals:						

VITAMINS/SUPPLEMENTS/MEDS.

Water: 1 2 3 4 5 6 7 8
(8 oz)

	Calories	Carbs (g)	Added Sugar (g)	Fiber (g)	Protein (g)	Fat (g)
DINNER						
Time: Totals:						
SNACK						
Time: Totals:						
Grand Totals:						

PHYSICAL ACTIVITY

Activity	Duration	Intensity	Cal/Burn

BLOOD SUGAR LOG

	Before	After	Insulin
Breakfast			
Lunch			
Dinner			
Bedtime			

NOTES:

Day: ⬚   ____/____/____   **Weight:** ⬚
(Date)

Sleep (hrs): 1 2 3 4 5 6 7 8

	Calories	Carbs (g)	Added Sugar (g)	Fiber (g)	Protein (g)	Fat (g)
BREAKFAST						
Time: Totals:						
SNACK						
Time: Totals:						
LUNCH						
Time: Totals:						
SNACK						
Time: Totals:						
Page Totals:						

VITAMINS/SUPPLEMENTS/MEDS.

Water: 1 2 3 4 5 6 7 8
(8 oz)

	Calories	Carbs (g)	Added Sugar (g)	Fiber (g)	Protein (g)	Fat (g)
DINNER						
Time: Totals:						
SNACK						
Time: Totals:						
Grand Totals:						

PHYSICAL ACTIVITY

Activity	Duration	Intensity	Cal/Burn

BLOOD SUGAR LOG

	Before	After	Insulin
Breakfast			
Lunch			
Dinner			
Bedtime			

NOTES:

Day: ☐   ____/____/____   Weight: ☐
(Date)

Sleep (hrs): 1 2 3 4 5 6 7 8

	Calories	Carbs (g)	Added Sugar (g)	Fiber (g)	Protein (g)	Fat (g)
BREAKFAST						
Time: Totals:						
SNACK						
Time: Totals:						
LUNCH						
Time: Totals:						
SNACK						
Time: Totals:						
Page Totals:						

VITAMINS/SUPPLEMENTS/MEDS.

Water: 1 2 3 4 5 6 7 8
(8 oz)

	Calories	Carbs (g)	Added Sugar (g)	Fiber (g)	Protein (g)	Fat (g)	
DINNER							
Time: Totals:							
SNACK							
Time: Totals:							
Grand Totals:							

PHYSICAL ACTIVITY

Activity	Duration	Intensity	Cal/Burn

BLOOD SUGAR LOG

	Before	After	Insulin
Breakfast			
Lunch			
Dinner			
Bedtime			

NOTES:

Day: [ ]　　　　____/____/____　　　　**Weight:** [ ]
(Date)

Sleep (hrs): 1 2 3 4 5 6 7 8

	Calories	Carbs (g)	Added Sugar (g)	Fiber (g)	Protein (g)	Fat (g)
BREAKFAST						
Time:　　　Totals:						
SNACK						
Time:　　　Totals:						
LUNCH						
Time:　　　Totals:						
SNACK						
Time:　　　Totals:						
Page Totals:						

VITAMINS/SUPPLEMENTS/MEDS.

Water: 1 2 3 4 5 6 7 8
(8 oz)

	Calories	Carbs (g)	Added Sugar (g)	Fiber (g)	Protein (g)	Fat (g)
DINNER						
Time:　　　　Totals:						
SNACK						
Time:　　　　Totals:						
Grand Totals:						

PHYSICAL ACTIVITY

Activity	Duration	Intensity	Cal/Burn

BLOOD SUGAR LOG

	Before	After	Insulin
Breakfast			
Lunch			
Dinner			
Bedtime			

NOTES:

Day: [ ]   ____/____/____   **Weight:** [ ]

(Date)

Sleep (hrs): 1 2 3 4 5 6 7 8

	Calories	Carbs (g)	Added Sugar (g)	Fiber (g)	Protein (g)	Fat (g)	
BREAKFAST							
Time: Totals:							
SNACK							
Time: Totals:							
LUNCH							
Time: Totals:							
SNACK							
Time: Totals:							
Page Totals:							

VITAMINS/SUPPLEMENTS/MEDS.

[ ]

Water: 1 2 3 4 5 6 7 8
(8 oz)

	Calories	Carbs (g)	Added Sugar (g)	Fiber (g)	Protein (g)	Fat (g)	
DINNER							
Time: Totals:							
SNACK							
Time: Totals:							
Grand Totals:							

PHYSICAL ACTIVITY

Activity	Duration	Intensity	Cal/Burn

BLOOD SUGAR LOG

	Before	After	Insulin
Breakfast			
Lunch			
Dinner			
Bedtime			

NOTES:

Day: ☐   ____/____/____   **Weight:** ☐
                                    (Date)

Sleep (hrs): 1 2 3 4 5 6 7 8

	Calories	Carbs (g)	Added Sugar (g)	Fiber (g)	Protein (g)	Fat (g)
BREAKFAST						
Time: Totals:						
SNACK						
Time: Totals:						
LUNCH						
Time: Totals:						
SNACK						
Time: Totals:						
Page Totals:						

VITAMINS/SUPPLEMENTS/MEDS.

Water: 1 2 3 4 5 6 7 8
(8 oz)

	Calories	Carbs (g)	Added Sugar (g)	Fiber (g)	Protein (g)	Fat (g)
DINNER						
Time: Totals:						
SNACK						
Time: Totals:						
Grand Totals:						

PHYSICAL ACTIVITY

Activity	Duration	Intensity	Cal/Burn

BLOOD SUGAR LOG

	Before	After	Insulin
Breakfast			
Lunch			
Dinner			
Bedtime			

NOTES:

Day: ☐ ____ / ____ / ____ **Weight:** ☐

(Date)

Sleep (hrs): 1 2 3 4 5 6 7 8

	Calories	Carbs (g)	Added Sugar (g)	Fiber (g)	Protein (g)	Fat (g)
BREAKFAST						
Time: Totals:						
SNACK						
Time: Totals:						
LUNCH						
Time: Totals:						
SNACK						
Time: Totals:						
Page Totals:						

VITAMINS/SUPPLEMENTS/MEDS.

Water: 1 2 3 4 5 6 7 8
(8 oz)

	Calories	Carbs (g)	Added Sugar (g)	Fiber (g)	Protein (g)	Fat (g)
DINNER						
Time: Totals:						
SNACK						
Time: Totals:						
Grand Totals:						

PHYSICAL ACTIVITY

Activity	Duration	Intensity	Cal/Burn

BLOOD SUGAR LOG

	Before	After	Insulin
Breakfast			
Lunch			
Dinner			
Bedtime			

NOTES:

_____
_____
_____
_____
_____

Day: ☐   _____/_____/_____   **Weight:** ☐
                    (Date)

Sleep (hrs): 1 2 3 4 5 6 7 8

	Calories	Carbs (g)	Added Sugar (g)	Fiber (g)	Protein (g)	Fat (g)
BREAKFAST						
Time: Totals:						
SNACK						
Time: Totals:						
LUNCH						
Time: Totals:						
SNACK						
Time: Totals:						
Page Totals:						

VITAMINS/SUPPLEMENTS/MEDS.

Water: 1 2 3 4 5 6 7 8
(8 oz)

	Calories	Carbs (g)	Added Sugar (g)	Fiber (g)	Protein (g)	Fat (g)	
DINNER							
Time: Totals:							
SNACK							
Time: Totals:							
Grand Totals:							

PHYSICAL ACTIVITY

Activity	Duration	Intensity	Cal/Burn

BLOOD SUGAR LOG

	Before	After	Insulin
Breakfast			
Lunch			
Dinner			
Bedtime			

NOTES:

Day: [ ] ____/____/____ Weight: [ ]
(Date)

Sleep (hrs): 1 2 3 4 5 6 7 8

	Calories	Carbs (g)	Added Sugar (g)	Fiber (g)	Protein (g)	Fat (g)
BREAKFAST						
Time: Totals:						
SNACK						
Time: Totals:						
LUNCH						
Time: Totals:						
SNACK						
Time: Totals:						
Page Totals:						

VITAMINS/SUPPLEMENTS/MEDS.

Water: 1 2 3 4 5 6 7 8
(8 oz)

	Calories	Carbs (g)	Added Sugar (g)	Fiber (g)	Protein (g)	Fat (g)
DINNER						
Time: Totals:						
SNACK						
Time: Totals:						
Grand Totals:						

PHYSICAL ACTIVITY

Activity	Duration	Intensity	Cal/Burn

BLOOD SUGAR LOG

	Before	After	Insulin
Breakfast			
Lunch			
Dinner			
Bedtime			

NOTES:

Day: ☐   ___/___/___   Weight: ☐

(Date)

Sleep (hrs): 1 2 3 4 5 6 7 8

	Calories	Carbs (g)	Added Sugar (g)	Fiber (g)	Protein (g)	Fat (g)
BREAKFAST						
Time: Totals:						
SNACK						
Time: Totals:						
LUNCH						
Time: Totals:						
SNACK						
Time: Totals:						
Page Totals:						

VITAMINS/SUPPLEMENTS/MEDS.

Water: 1 2 3 4 5 6 7 8
(8 oz)

	Calories	Carbs (g)	Added Sugar (g)	Fiber (g)	Protein (g)	Fat (g)
DINNER						
Time: Totals:						
SNACK						
Time: Totals:						
Grand Totals:						

PHYSICAL ACTIVITY

Activity	Duration	Intensity	Cal/Burn

BLOOD SUGAR LOG

	Before	After	Insulin
Breakfast			
Lunch			
Dinner			
Bedtime			

NOTES:

Day: ☐   ____/____/____   Weight: ☐

(Date)

Sleep (hrs): 1 2 3 4 5 6 7 8

	Calories	Carbs (g)	Added Sugar (g)	Fiber (g)	Protein (g)	Fat (g)	
BREAKFAST							
Time: Totals:							
SNACK							
Time: Totals:							
LUNCH							
Time: Totals:							
SNACK							
Time: Totals:							
Page Totals:							

VITAMINS/SUPPLEMENTS/MEDS.

Water: 1 2 3 4 5 6 7 8
(8 oz)

	Calories	Carbs (g)	Added Sugar (g)	Fiber (g)	Protein (g)	Fat (g)	
DINNER							
Time: Totals:							
SNACK							
Time: Totals:							
Grand Totals:							

PHYSICAL ACTIVITY

Activity	Duration	Intensity	Cal/Burn

BLOOD SUGAR LOG

	Before	After	Insulin
Breakfast			
Lunch			
Dinner			
Bedtime			

NOTES:

Day: ☐   ____/____/____   Weight: ☐
                  (Date)

Sleep (hrs): 1 2 3 4 5 6 7 8

	Calories	Carbs (g)	Added Sugar (g)	Fiber (g)	Protein (g)	Fat (g)
BREAKFAST						
Time: Totals:						
SNACK						
Time: Totals:						
LUNCH						
Time: Totals:						
SNACK						
Time: Totals:						
Page Totals:						

VITAMINS/SUPPLEMENTS/MEDS.

Water: 1 2 3 4 5 6 7 8
(8 oz)

	Calories	Carbs (g)	Added Sugar (g)	Fiber (g)	Protein (g)	Fat (g)
DINNER						
Time: Totals:						
SNACK						
Time: Totals:						
Grand Totals:						

PHYSICAL ACTIVITY

Activity	Duration	Intensity	Cal/Burn

BLOOD SUGAR LOG

	Before	After	Insulin
Breakfast			
Lunch			
Dinner			
Bedtime			

NOTES:

Day: ☐   _____ / _____ / _____   **Weight:** ☐
(Date)

Sleep (hrs): 1 2 3 4 5 6 7 8

	Calories	Carbs (g)	Added Sugar (g)	Fiber (g)	Protein (g)	Fat (g)
BREAKFAST						
Time: Totals:						
SNACK						
Time: Totals:						
LUNCH						
Time: Totals:						
SNACK						
Time: Totals:						
Page Totals:						

VITAMINS/SUPPLEMENTS/MEDS.

Water: 1 2 3 4 5 6 7 8
(8 oz)

	Calories	Carbs (g)	Added Sugar (g)	Fiber (g)	Protein (g)	Fat (g)
DINNER						
Time: Totals:						
SNACK						
Time: Totals:						
Grand Totals:						

PHYSICAL ACTIVITY

Activity	Duration	Intensity	Cal/Burn

BLOOD SUGAR LOG

	Before	After	Insulin
Breakfast			
Lunch			
Dinner			
Bedtime			

NOTES:

Day: ☐   ____/____/____
(Date)   **Weight:** ☐

Sleep (hrs): 1 2 3 4 5 6 7 8

	Calories	Carbs (g)	Added Sugar (g)	Fiber (g)	Protein (g)	Fat (g)
BREAKFAST						
Time: Totals:						
SNACK						
Time: Totals:						
LUNCH						
Time: Totals:						
SNACK						
Time: Totals:						
Page Totals:						

VITAMINS/SUPPLEMENTS/MEDS.

Water: 1 2 3 4 5 6 7 8
(8 oz)

	Calories	Carbs (g)	Added Sugar (g)	Fiber (g)	Protein (g)	Fat (g)	
DINNER							
Time: Totals:							
SNACK							
Time: Totals:							
Grand Totals:							

PHYSICAL ACTIVITY

Activity	Duration	Intensity	Cal/Burn

BLOOD SUGAR LOG

	Before	After	Insulin
Breakfast			
Lunch			
Dinner			
Bedtime			

NOTES:

Day: ⬜   ____/____/____   **Weight:** ⬜
                           (Date)

Sleep (hrs): 1 2 3 4 5 6 7 8

	Calories	Carbs (g)	Added Sugar (g)	Fiber (g)	Protein (g)	Fat (g)
BREAKFAST						
Time: Totals:						
SNACK						
Time: Totals:						
LUNCH						
Time: Totals:						
SNACK						
Time: Totals:						
Page Totals:						

VITAMINS/SUPPLEMENTS/MEDS.

Water: 1 2 3 4 5 6 7 8
(8 oz)

	Calories	Carbs (g)	Added Sugar (g)	Fiber (g)	Protein (g)	Fat (g)
DINNER						
Time: Totals:						
SNACK						
Time: Totals:						
Grand Totals:						

PHYSICAL ACTIVITY

Activity	Duration	Intensity	Cal/Burn

BLOOD SUGAR LOG

	Before	After	Insulin
Breakfast			
Lunch			
Dinner			
Bedtime			

NOTES:

Day: [ ] ____/____/____ Weight: [ ]
(Date)

Sleep (hrs): 1 2 3 4 5 6 7 8

	Calories	Carbs (g)	Added Sugar (g)	Fiber (g)	Protein (g)	Fat (g)
BREAKFAST						
Time: Totals:						
SNACK						
Time: Totals:						
LUNCH						
Time: Totals:						
SNACK						
Time: Totals:						
Page Totals:						

VITAMINS/SUPPLEMENTS/MEDS.

Water: 1 2 3 4 5 6 7 8
(8 oz)

	Calories	Carbs (g)	Added Sugar (g)	Fiber (g)	Protein (g)	Fat (g)
DINNER						
Time: Totals:						
SNACK						
Time: Totals:						
Grand Totals:						

PHYSICAL ACTIVITY

Activity	Duration	Intensity	Cal/Burn

BLOOD SUGAR LOG

	Before	After	Insulin
Breakfast			
Lunch			
Dinner			
Bedtime			

NOTES:

_____
_____
_____
_____
_____

Day: ☐   _____ / _____ / _____   **Weight:** ☐

(Date)

Sleep (hrs): 1 2 3 4 5 6 7 8

	Calories	Carbs (g)	Added Sugar (g)	Fiber (g)	Protein (g)	Fat (g)
BREAKFAST						
Time: Totals:						
SNACK						
Time: Totals:						
LUNCH						
Time: Totals:						
SNACK						
Time: Totals:						
Page Totals:						

VITAMINS/SUPPLEMENTS/MEDS.

Water: 1 2 3 4 5 6 7 8
(8 oz)

	Calories	Carbs (g)	Added Sugar (g)	Fiber (g)	Protein (g)	Fat (g)	
DINNER							
Time: Totals:							
SNACK							
Time: Totals:							
Grand Totals:							

PHYSICAL ACTIVITY

Activity	Duration	Intensity	Cal/Burn

BLOOD SUGAR LOG

	Before	After	Insulin
Breakfast			
Lunch			
Dinner			
Bedtime			

NOTES:

Day: ☐   ____/____/____   **Weight:** ☐

(Date)

Sleep (hrs): 1 2 3 4 5 6 7 8

	Calories	Carbs (g)	Added Sugar (g)	Fiber (g)	Protein (g)	Fat (g)
BREAKFAST						
Time: Totals:						
SNACK						
Time: Totals:						
LUNCH						
Time: Totals:						
SNACK						
Time: Totals:						
Page Totals:						

VITAMINS/SUPPLEMENTS/MEDS.

Water: 1 2 3 4 5 6 7 8
(8 oz)

	Calories	Carbs (g)	Added Sugar (g)	Fiber (g)	Protein (g)	Fat (g)
DINNER						
Time: Totals:						
SNACK						
Time: Totals:						
Grand Totals:						

PHYSICAL ACTIVITY

Activity	Duration	Intensity	Cal/Burn

BLOOD SUGAR LOG

	Before	After	Insulin
Breakfast			
Lunch			
Dinner			
Bedtime			

NOTES:

Day: [　　　]　　　　　___/___/___　　　Weight: [　　　]
　　　　　　　　　　　　　　(Date)

Sleep (hrs): 1 2 3 4 5 6 7 8

	Calories	Carbs (g)	Added Sugar (g)	Fiber (g)	Protein (g)	Fat (g)
BREAKFAST						
Time:　　　　Totals:						
SNACK						
Time:　　　　Totals:						
LUNCH						
Time:　　　　Totals:						
SNACK						
Time:　　　　Totals:						
Page Totals:						

VITAMINS/SUPPLEMENTS/MEDS.

[　　　　　　　　　　　　　　　　　　　　　　　]

Water: 1 2 3 4 5 6 7 8
(8 oz)

	Calories	Carbs (g)	Added Sugar (g)	Fiber (g)	Protein (g)	Fat (g)
DINNER						
Time:　　　Totals:						
SNACK						
Time:　　　Totals:						
Grand Totals:						

PHYSICAL ACTIVITY

Activity	Duration	Intensity	Cal/Burn

BLOOD SUGAR LOG

	Before	After	Insulin
Breakfast			
Lunch			
Dinner			
Bedtime			

NOTES:

Day: [ ]   ____/____/____   Weight: [ ]
                  (Date)

Sleep (hrs): 1 2 3 4 5 6 7 8

	Calories	Carbs (g)	Added Sugar (g)	Fiber (g)	Protein (g)	Fat (g)
BREAKFAST						
Time: Totals:						
SNACK						
Time: Totals:						
LUNCH						
Time: Totals:						
SNACK						
Time: Totals:						
Page Totals:						

VITAMINS/SUPPLEMENTS/MEDS.

Water: 1 2 3 4 5 6 7 8
(8 oz)

	Calories	Carbs (g)	Added Sugar (g)	Fiber (g)	Protein (g)	Fat (g)
DINNER						
Time: Totals:						
SNACK						
Time: Totals:						
Grand Totals:						

PHYSICAL ACTIVITY

Activity	Duration	Intensity	Cal/Burn

BLOOD SUGAR LOG

	Before	After	Insulin
Breakfast			
Lunch			
Dinner			
Bedtime			

NOTES:

_____
_____
_____
_____
_____

Day: [ ]   ____ / ____ / ____   **Weight:** [ ]

(Date)

Sleep (hrs): 1 2 3 4 5 6 7 8

	Calories	Carbs (g)	Added Sugar (g)	Fiber (g)	Protein (g)	Fat (g)
BREAKFAST						
Time: Totals:						
SNACK						
Time: Totals:						
LUNCH						
Time: Totals:						
SNACK						
Time: Totals:						
Page Totals:						

VITAMINS/SUPPLEMENTS/MEDS.

Water: 1 2 3 4 5 6 7 8
(8 oz)

	Calories	Carbs (g)	Added Sugar (g)	Fiber (g)	Protein (g)	Fat (g)
DINNER						
Time: Totals:						
SNACK						
Time: Totals:						
Grand Totals:						

PHYSICAL ACTIVITY

Activity	Duration	Intensity	Cal/Burn

BLOOD SUGAR LOG

	Before	After	Insulin
Breakfast			
Lunch			
Dinner			
Bedtime			

NOTES:

Day: ☐   _____ / _____ / _____   **Weight:** ☐
(Date)

Sleep (hrs): 1 2 3 4 5 6 7 8

	Calories	Carbs (g)	Added Sugar (g)	Fiber (g)	Protein (g)	Fat (g)
BREAKFAST						
Time: Totals:						
SNACK						
Time: Totals:						
LUNCH						
Time: Totals:						
SNACK						
Time: Totals:						
Page Totals:						

VITAMINS/SUPPLEMENTS/MEDS.

Water: 1 2 3 4 5 6 7 8
(8 oz)

	Calories	Carbs (g)	Added Sugar (g)	Fiber (g)	Protein (g)	Fat (g)	
DINNER							
Time: Totals:							
SNACK							
Time: Totals:							
Grand Totals:							

PHYSICAL ACTIVITY

Activity	Duration	Intensity	Cal/Burn

BLOOD SUGAR LOG

	Before	After	Insulin
Breakfast			
Lunch			
Dinner			
Bedtime			

NOTES:

___
___
___
___

Day: [ ]　　　　____/____/____　　　**Weight:** [ ]
　　　　　　　　　　　　(Date)

Sleep (hrs): 1 2 3 4 5 6 7 8

	Calories	Carbs (g)	Added Sugar (g)	Fiber (g)	Protein (g)	Fat (g)
BREAKFAST						
Time:　　Totals:						
SNACK						
Time:　　Totals:						
LUNCH						
Time:　　Totals:						
SNACK						
Time:　　Totals:						
Page Totals:						

VITAMINS/SUPPLEMENTS/MEDS.

[ ]

Water: 1 2 3 4 5 6 7 8
(8 oz)

	Calories	Carbs (g)	Added Sugar (g)	Fiber (g)	Protein (g)	Fat (g)	
DINNER							
Time: Totals:							
SNACK							
Time: Totals:							
Grand Totals:							

PHYSICAL ACTIVITY

Activity	Duration	Intensity	Cal/Burn

BLOOD SUGAR LOG

	Before	After	Insulin
Breakfast			
Lunch			
Dinner			
Bedtime			

NOTES:

Day: [ ]   ____/____/____   Weight: [ ]
(Date)

Sleep (hrs): 1 2 3 4 5 6 7 8

	Calories	Carbs (g)	Added Sugar (g)	Fiber (g)	Protein (g)	Fat (g)
BREAKFAST						
Time: Totals:						
SNACK						
Time: Totals:						
LUNCH						
Time: Totals:						
SNACK						
Time: Totals:						
Page Totals:						

VITAMINS/SUPPLEMENTS/MEDS.

Water: 1 2 3 4 5 6 7 8
(8 oz)

	Calories	Carbs (g)	Added Sugar (g)	Fiber (g)	Protein (g)	Fat (g)
DINNER						
Time: Totals:						
SNACK						
Time: Totals:						
Grand Totals:						

PHYSICAL ACTIVITY

Activity	Duration	Intensity	Cal/Burn

BLOOD SUGAR LOG

	Before	After	Insulin
Breakfast			
Lunch			
Dinner			
Bedtime			

NOTES:

Day: ☐   ____/____/____   Weight: ☐
                    (Date)

Sleep (hrs): 1 2 3 4 5 6 7 8

	Calories	Carbs (g)	Added Sugar (g)	Fiber (g)	Protein (g)	Fat (g)
BREAKFAST						
Time: Totals:						
SNACK						
Time: Totals:						
LUNCH						
Time: Totals:						
SNACK						
Time: Totals:						
Page Totals:						

VITAMINS/SUPPLEMENTS/MEDS.

Water: 1 2 3 4 5 6 7 8
(8 oz)

	Calories	Carbs (g)	Added Sugar (g)	Fiber (g)	Protein (g)	Fat (g)
DINNER						
Time: Totals:						
SNACK						
Time: Totals:						
Grand Totals:						

PHYSICAL ACTIVITY

Activity	Duration	Intensity	Cal/Burn

BLOOD SUGAR LOG

	Before	After	Insulin
Breakfast			
Lunch			
Dinner			
Bedtime			

NOTES:

Day: ☐   ____/____/____   **Weight:** ☐
(Date)

Sleep (hrs): 1 2 3 4 5 6 7 8

	Calories	Carbs (g)	Added Sugar (g)	Fiber (g)	Protein (g)	Fat (g)
BREAKFAST						
Time: Totals:						
SNACK						
Time: Totals:						
LUNCH						
Time: Totals:						
SNACK						
Time: Totals:						
Page Totals:						

VITAMINS/SUPPLEMENTS/MEDS.

Water: 1 2 3 4 5 6 7 8
(8 oz)

	Calories	Carbs (g)	Added Sugar (g)	Fiber (g)	Protein (g)	Fat (g)
DINNER						
Time: Totals:						
SNACK						
Time: Totals:						
Grand Totals:						

PHYSICAL ACTIVITY

Activity	Duration	Intensity	Cal/Burn

BLOOD SUGAR LOG

	Before	After	Insulin
Breakfast			
Lunch			
Dinner			
Bedtime			

NOTES:

Day: [ ]   ____ / ____ / ____   Weight: [ ]
                     (Date)

Sleep (hrs): 1 2 3 4 5 6 7 8

	Calories	Carbs (g)	Added Sugar (g)	Fiber (g)	Protein (g)	Fat (g)
BREAKFAST						
Time: Totals:						
SNACK						
Time: Totals:						
LUNCH						
Time: Totals:						
SNACK						
Time: Totals:						
Page Totals:						

VITAMINS/SUPPLEMENTS/MEDS.

[ ]

Water: 1 2 3 4 5 6 7 8
(8 oz)

	Calories	Carbs (g)	Added Sugar (g)	Fiber (g)	Protein (g)	Fat (g)	
DINNER							
Time: Totals:							
SNACK							
Time: Totals:							
Grand Totals:							

PHYSICAL ACTIVITY

Activity	Duration	Intensity	Cal/Burn

BLOOD SUGAR LOG

	Before	After	Insulin
Breakfast			
Lunch			
Dinner			
Bedtime			

NOTES:

Day: [ ] ____/____/_____
(Date)
Weight: [ ]

Sleep (hrs): 1 2 3 4 5 6 7 8

	Calories	Carbs (g)	Added Sugar (g)	Fiber (g)	Protein (g)	Fat (g)
BREAKFAST						
Time: Totals:						
SNACK						
Time: Totals:						
LUNCH						
Time: Totals:						
SNACK						
Time: Totals:						
Page Totals:						

VITAMINS/SUPPLEMENTS/MEDS.

[ ]

Water: 1 2 3 4 5 6 7 8
(8 oz)

	Calories	Carbs (g)	Added Sugar (g)	Fiber (g)	Protein (g)	Fat (g)
DINNER						
Time: Totals:						
SNACK						
Time: Totals:						
Grand Totals:						

PHYSICAL ACTIVITY

Activity	Duration	Intensity	Cal/Burn

BLOOD SUGAR LOG

	Before	After	Insulin
Breakfast			
Lunch			
Dinner			
Bedtime			

NOTES:

Day: ☐   _____/_____/_____   **Weight:** ☐
(Date)

Sleep (hrs): 1 2 3 4 5 6 7 8

	Calories	Carbs (g)	Added Sugar (g)	Fiber (g)	Protein (g)	Fat (g)
BREAKFAST						
Time: Totals:						
SNACK						
Time: Totals:						
LUNCH						
Time: Totals:						
SNACK						
Time: Totals:						
Page Totals:						

VITAMINS/SUPPLEMENTS/MEDS.

Water: 1 2 3 4 5 6 7 8
(8 oz)

	Calories	Carbs (g)	Added Sugar (g)	Fiber (g)	Protein (g)	Fat (g)	
DINNER							
Time: Totals:							
SNACK							
Time: Totals:							
Grand Totals:							

PHYSICAL ACTIVITY

Activity	Duration	Intensity	Cal/Burn

BLOOD SUGAR LOG

	Before	After	Insulin
Breakfast			
Lunch			
Dinner			
Bedtime			

NOTES:

Day: [ ]   ____/____/____   **Weight:** [ ]

(Date)

Sleep (hrs): 1 2 3 4 5 6 7 8

	Calories	Carbs (g)	Added Sugar (g)	Fiber (g)	Protein (g)	Fat (g)
BREAKFAST						
Time: Totals:						
SNACK						
Time: Totals:						
LUNCH						
Time: Totals:						
SNACK						
Time: Totals:						
Page Totals:						

VITAMINS/SUPPLEMENTS/MEDS.

Water: 1 2 3 4 5 6 7 8
(8 oz)

	Calories	Carbs (g)	Added Sugar (g)	Fiber (g)	Protein (g)	Fat (g)
DINNER						
Time: Totals:						
SNACK						
Time: Totals:						
Grand Totals:						

PHYSICAL ACTIVITY

Activity	Duration	Intensity	Cal/Burn

BLOOD SUGAR LOG

	Before	After	Insulin
Breakfast			
Lunch			
Dinner			
Bedtime			

NOTES:

Day: ☐   ____/____/____   Weight: ☐
                  (Date)

Sleep (hrs): 1 2 3 4 5 6 7 8

	Calories	Carbs (g)	Added Sugar (g)	Fiber (g)	Protein (g)	Fat (g)
BREAKFAST						
Time: Totals:						
SNACK						
Time: Totals:						
LUNCH						
Time: Totals:						
SNACK						
Time: Totals:						
Page Totals:						

VITAMINS/SUPPLEMENTS/MEDS.

Water: 1 2 3 4 5 6 7 8
(8 oz)

	Calories	Carbs (g)	Added Sugar (g)	Fiber (g)	Protein (g)	Fat (g)
DINNER						
Time: Totals:						
SNACK						
Time: Totals:						
Grand Totals:						

PHYSICAL ACTIVITY

Activity	Duration	Intensity	Cal/Burn

BLOOD SUGAR LOG

	Before	After	Insulin
Breakfast			
Lunch			
Dinner			
Bedtime			

NOTES:

Day: [ ]　　　　____/____/____　　　　**Weight:** [ ]
　　　　　　　　　　　　(Date)

Sleep (hrs): 1 2 3 4 5 6 7 8

	Calories	Carbs (g)	Added Sugar (g)	Fiber (g)	Protein (g)	Fat (g)
BREAKFAST						
Time:　　　Totals:						
SNACK						
Time:　　　Totals:						
LUNCH						
Time:　　　Totals:						
SNACK						
Time:　　　Totals:						
Page Totals:						

VITAMINS/SUPPLEMENTS/MEDS.

[ ]

Water: 1 2 3 4 5 6 7 8
(8 oz)

	Calories	Carbs (g)	Added Sugar (g)	Fiber (g)	Protein (g)	Fat (g)
DINNER						
Time: Totals:						
SNACK						
Time: Totals:						
Grand Totals:						

PHYSICAL ACTIVITY

Activity	Duration	Intensity	Cal/Burn

BLOOD SUGAR LOG

	Before	After	Insulin
Breakfast			
Lunch			
Dinner			
Bedtime			

NOTES:

Day: [ ] _____ / _____ / _____ Weight: [ ]
(Date)

Sleep (hrs): 1 2 3 4 5 6 7 8

	Calories	Carbs (g)	Added Sugar (g)	Fiber (g)	Protein (g)	Fat (g)
BREAKFAST						
Time: Totals:						
SNACK						
Time: Totals:						
LUNCH						
Time: Totals:						
SNACK						
Time: Totals:						
Page Totals:						

VITAMINS/SUPPLEMENTS/MEDS.

Water: 1 2 3 4 5 6 7 8
(8 oz)

	Calories	Carbs (g)	Added Sugar (g)	Fiber (g)	Protein (g)	Fat (g)
DINNER						
Time: Totals:						
SNACK						
Time: Totals:						
Grand Totals:						

PHYSICAL ACTIVITY

Activity	Duration	Intensity	Cal/Burn

BLOOD SUGAR LOG

	Before	After	Insulin
Breakfast			
Lunch			
Dinner			
Bedtime			

NOTES:

Day: [ ]   ____ / ____ / ____   Weight: [ ]

(Date)

Sleep (hrs): 1 2 3 4 5 6 7 8

	Calories	Carbs (g)	Added Sugar (g)	Fiber (g)	Protein (g)	Fat (g)
BREAKFAST						
Time: Totals:						
SNACK						
Time: Totals:						
LUNCH						
Time: Totals:						
SNACK						
Time: Totals:						
Page Totals:						

VITAMINS/SUPPLEMENTS/MEDS.

Water: 1 2 3 4 5 6 7 8
(8 oz)

	Calories	Carbs (g)	Added Sugar (g)	Fiber (g)	Protein (g)	Fat (g)
DINNER						
Time: Totals:						
SNACK						
Time: Totals:						
Grand Totals:						

PHYSICAL ACTIVITY

Activity	Duration	Intensity	Cal/Burn

BLOOD SUGAR LOG

	Before	After	Insulin
Breakfast			
Lunch			
Dinner			
Bedtime			

NOTES:

Day: [ ] _____/_____/_____ Weight: [ ]
(Date)

Sleep (hrs): 1 2 3 4 5 6 7 8

	Calories	Carbs (g)	Added Sugar (g)	Fiber (g)	Protein (g)	Fat (g)
BREAKFAST						
Time: Totals:						
SNACK						
Time: Totals:						
LUNCH						
Time: Totals:						
SNACK						
Time: Totals:						
Page Totals:						

VITAMINS/SUPPLEMENTS/MEDS.

Water: 1 2 3 4 5 6 7 8
(8 oz)

	Calories	Carbs (g)	Added Sugar (g)	Fiber (g)	Protein (g)	Fat (g)
DINNER						
Time: Totals:						
SNACK						
Time: Totals:						
Grand Totals:						

PHYSICAL ACTIVITY

Activity	Duration	Intensity	Cal/Burn

BLOOD SUGAR LOG

	Before	After	Insulin
Breakfast			
Lunch			
Dinner			
Bedtime			

NOTES:

Day: [ ]   ____/____/____   **Weight:** [ ]

(Date)

Sleep (hrs): 1 2 3 4 5 6 7 8

	Calories	Carbs (g)	Added Sugar (g)	Fiber (g)	Protein (g)	Fat (g)
BREAKFAST						
Time: Totals:						
SNACK						
Time: Totals:						
LUNCH						
Time: Totals:						
SNACK						
Time: Totals:						
Page Totals:						

VITAMINS/SUPPLEMENTS/MEDS.

Water: 1 2 3 4 5 6 7 8
(8 oz)

	Calories	Carbs (g)	Added Sugar (g)	Fiber (g)	Protein (g)	Fat (g)
DINNER						
Time: Totals:						
SNACK						
Time: Totals:						
Grand Totals:						

PHYSICAL ACTIVITY

Activity	Duration	Intensity	Cal/Burn

BLOOD SUGAR LOG

	Before	After	Insulin
Breakfast			
Lunch			
Dinner			
Bedtime			

NOTES:

Day: [ ]   ____/____/____   Weight: [ ]
                     (Date)

Sleep (hrs): 1 2 3 4 5 6 7 8

	Calories	Carbs (g)	Added Sugar (g)	Fiber (g)	Protein (g)	Fat (g)
BREAKFAST						
Time: Totals:						
SNACK						
Time: Totals:						
LUNCH						
Time: Totals:						
SNACK						
Time: Totals:						
Page Totals:						

VITAMINS/SUPPLEMENTS/MEDS.

Water: 1 2 3 4 5 6 7 8
(8 oz)

	Calories	Carbs (g)	Added Sugar (g)	Fiber (g)	Protein (g)	Fat (g)
DINNER						
Time: Totals:						
SNACK						
Time: Totals:						
Grand Totals:						

PHYSICAL ACTIVITY

Activity	Duration	Intensity	Cal/Burn

BLOOD SUGAR LOG

	Before	After	Insulin
Breakfast			
Lunch			
Dinner			
Bedtime			

NOTES:

Day: ☐   ____/____/____   **Weight:** ☐
                    (Date)

Sleep (hrs): 1 2 3 4 5 6 7 8

	Calories	Carbs (g)	Added Sugar (g)	Fiber (g)	Protein (g)	Fat (g)
BREAKFAST						
Time: Totals:						
SNACK						
Time: Totals:						
LUNCH						
Time: Totals:						
SNACK						
Time: Totals:						
Page Totals:						

VITAMINS/SUPPLEMENTS/MEDS.

Water: 1 2 3 4 5 6 7 8
(8 oz)

	Calories	Carbs (g)	Added Sugar (g)	Fiber (g)	Protein (g)	Fat (g)
DINNER						
Time: Totals:						
SNACK						
Time: Totals:						
Grand Totals:						

PHYSICAL ACTIVITY

Activity	Duration	Intensity	Cal/Burn

BLOOD SUGAR LOG

	Before	After	Insulin
Breakfast			
Lunch			
Dinner			
Bedtime			

NOTES:

Day: [   ]   ____/____/____   Weight: [   ]
                          (Date)

Sleep (hrs): 1 2 3 4 5 6 7 8

	Calories	Carbs (g)	Added Sugar (g)	Fiber (g)	Protein (g)	Fat (g)
BREAKFAST						
Time: Totals:						
SNACK						
Time: Totals:						
LUNCH						
Time: Totals:						
SNACK						
Time: Totals:						
Page Totals:						

VITAMINS/SUPPLEMENTS/MEDS.

[   ]

Water: 1 2 3 4 5 6 7 8
(8 oz)

	Calories	Carbs (g)	Added Sugar (g)	Fiber (g)	Protein (g)	Fat (g)
DINNER						
Time: Totals:						
SNACK						
Time: Totals:						
Grand Totals:						

PHYSICAL ACTIVITY

Activity	Duration	Intensity	Cal/Burn

BLOOD SUGAR LOG

	Before	After	Insulin
Breakfast			
Lunch			
Dinner			
Bedtime			

NOTES:

Day: ☐   ___/___/___   **Weight:** ☐
(Date)

Sleep (hrs): 1 2 3 4 5 6 7 8

	Calories	Carbs (g)	Added Sugar (g)	Fiber (g)	Protein (g)	Fat (g)
BREAKFAST						
Time: Totals:						
SNACK						
Time: Totals:						
LUNCH						
Time: Totals:						
SNACK						
Time: Totals:						
Page Totals:						

VITAMINS/SUPPLEMENTS/MEDS.

Water: 1 2 3 4 5 6 7 8
(8 oz)

DINNER	Calories	Carbs (g)	Added Sugar (g)	Fiber (g)	Protein (g)	Fat (g)
Time: Totals:						
SNACK						
Time: Totals:						
Grand Totals:						

PHYSICAL ACTIVITY

Activity	Duration	Intensity	Cal/Burn

BLOOD SUGAR LOG

	Before	After	Insulin
Breakfast			
Lunch			
Dinner			
Bedtime			

NOTES:

_____
_____
_____
_____
_____

Day: [ ] ____/____/____ **Weight:** [   ]
(Date)

Sleep (hrs): 1 2 3 4 5 6 7 8

	Calories	Carbs (g)	Added Sugar (g)	Fiber (g)	Protein (g)	Fat (g)
BREAKFAST						
Time: Totals:						
SNACK						
Time: Totals:						
LUNCH						
Time: Totals:						
SNACK						
Time: Totals:						
Page Totals:						

VITAMINS/SUPPLEMENTS/MEDS.

[   ]

Water: 1 2 3 4 5 6 7 8
(8 oz)

	Calories	Carbs (g)	Added Sugar (g)	Fiber (g)	Protein (g)	Fat (g)
DINNER						
Time: Totals:						
SNACK						
Time: Totals:						
Grand Totals:						

PHYSICAL ACTIVITY

Activity	Duration	Intensity	Cal/Burn

BLOOD SUGAR LOG

	Before	After	Insulin
Breakfast			
Lunch			
Dinner			
Bedtime			

NOTES:

Day: ⬜   ____ / ____ / ____   Weight: ⬜

(Date)

Sleep (hrs): 1 2 3 4 5 6 7 8

	Calories	Carbs (g)	Added Sugar (g)	Fiber (g)	Protein (g)	Fat (g)
BREAKFAST						
Time: Totals:						
SNACK						
Time: Totals:						
LUNCH						
Time: Totals:						
SNACK						
Time: Totals:						
Page Totals:						

VITAMINS/SUPPLEMENTS/MEDS.

Water: 1 2 3 4 5 6 7 8
(8 oz)

	Calories	Carbs (g)	Added Sugar (g)	Fiber (g)	Protein (g)	Fat (g)
DINNER						
Time: Totals:						
SNACK						
Time: Totals:						
Grand Totals:						

PHYSICAL ACTIVITY

Activity	Duration	Intensity	Cal/Burn

BLOOD SUGAR LOG

	Before	After	Insulin
Breakfast			
Lunch			
Dinner			
Bedtime			

NOTES:

Day: ____   ____/____/____   Weight: _____
                 (Date)

Sleep (hrs): 1 2 3 4 5 6 7 8

	Calories	Carbs (g)	Added Sugar (g)	Fiber (g)	Protein (g)	Fat (g)
BREAKFAST						
Time: Totals:						
SNACK						
Time: Totals:						
LUNCH						
Time: Totals:						
SNACK						
Time: Totals:						
Page Totals:						

VITAMINS/SUPPLEMENTS/MEDS.

Water: 1 2 3 4 5 6 7 8
(8 oz)

	Calories	Carbs (g)	Added Sugar (g)	Fiber (g)	Protein (g)	Fat (g)	
DINNER							
Time: Totals:							
SNACK							
Time: Totals:							
Grand Totals:							

PHYSICAL ACTIVITY

Activity	Duration	Intensity	Cal/Burn

BLOOD SUGAR LOG

	Before	After	Insulin
Breakfast			
Lunch			
Dinner			
Bedtime			

NOTES:

Day: [ ]   ____/____/____   Weight: [ ]
                      (Date)

Sleep (hrs): 1 2 3 4 5 6 7 8

	Calories	Carbs (g)	Added Sugar (g)	Fiber (g)	Protein (g)	Fat (g)
BREAKFAST						
Time: Totals:						
SNACK						
Time: Totals:						
LUNCH						
Time: Totals:						
SNACK						
Time: Totals:						
Page Totals:						

VITAMINS/SUPPLEMENTS/MEDS.

Water: 1 2 3 4 5 6 7 8
(8 oz)

	Calories	Carbs (g)	Added Sugar (g)	Fiber (g)	Protein (g)	Fat (g)
DINNER						
Time: Totals:						
SNACK						
Time: Totals:						
Grand Totals:						

PHYSICAL ACTIVITY

Activity	Duration	Intensity	Cal/Burn

BLOOD SUGAR LOG

	Before	After	Insulin
Breakfast			
Lunch			
Dinner			
Bedtime			

NOTES:

Day: [ ]   ____/____/____   Weight: [ ]

(Date)

Sleep (hrs): 1 2 3 4 5 6 7 8

	Calories	Carbs (g)	Added Sugar (g)	Fiber (g)	Protein (g)	Fat (g)
BREAKFAST						
Time: Totals:						
SNACK						
Time: Totals:						
LUNCH						
Time: Totals:						
SNACK						
Time: Totals:						
Page Totals:						

VITAMINS/SUPPLEMENTS/MEDS.

Water: 1 2 3 4 5 6 7 8
(8 oz)

	Calories	Carbs (g)	Added Sugar (g)	Fiber (g)	Protein (g)	Fat (g)
DINNER						
Time: Totals:						
SNACK						
Time: Totals:						
Grand Totals:						

PHYSICAL ACTIVITY

Activity	Duration	Intensity	Cal/Burn

BLOOD SUGAR LOG

	Before	After	Insulin
Breakfast			
Lunch			
Dinner			
Bedtime			

NOTES:

Day: [ ]　　　　　____ / ____ / ____　　　　　Weight: [ ]
(Date)

Sleep (hrs): 1 2 3 4 5 6 7 8

	Calories	Carbs (g)	Added Sugar (g)	Fiber (g)	Protein (g)	Fat (g)
BREAKFAST						
Time:　　　Totals:						
SNACK						
Time:　　　Totals:						
LUNCH						
Time:　　　Totals:						
SNACK						
Time:　　　Totals:						
Page Totals:						

VITAMINS/SUPPLEMENTS/MEDS.

Water: 1 2 3 4 5 6 7 8
(8 oz)

	Calories	Carbs (g)	Added Sugar (g)	Fiber (g)	Protein (g)	Fat (g)
DINNER						
Time: Totals:						
SNACK						
Time: Totals:						
Grand Totals:						

PHYSICAL ACTIVITY

Activity	Duration	Intensity	Cal/Burn

BLOOD SUGAR LOG

	Before	After	Insulin
Breakfast			
Lunch			
Dinner			
Bedtime			

NOTES:

Day: [ ]   ____/____/____   Weight: [ ]
                    (Date)

Sleep (hrs): 1 2 3 4 5 6 7 8

	Calories	Carbs (g)	Added Sugar (g)	Fiber (g)	Protein (g)	Fat (g)
BREAKFAST						
Time: Totals:						
SNACK						
Time: Totals:						
LUNCH						
Time: Totals:						
SNACK						
Time: Totals:						
Page Totals:						

VITAMINS/SUPPLEMENTS/MEDS.

Water: 1 2 3 4 5 6 7 8
(8 oz)

	Calories	Carbs (g)	Added Sugar (g)	Fiber (g)	Protein (g)	Fat (g)
DINNER						
Time: Totals:						
SNACK						
Time: Totals:						
Grand Totals:						

PHYSICAL ACTIVITY

Activity	Duration	Intensity	Cal/Burn

BLOOD SUGAR LOG

	Before	After	Insulin
Breakfast			
Lunch			
Dinner			
Bedtime			

NOTES:

Day: [ ]   ___ / ___ / ___   Weight: [ ]
                      (Date)

Sleep (hrs): 1 2 3 4 5 6 7 8

	Calories	Carbs (g)	Added Sugar (g)	Fiber (g)	Protein (g)	Fat (g)
BREAKFAST						
Time: Totals:						
SNACK						
Time: Totals:						
LUNCH						
Time: Totals:						
SNACK						
Time: Totals:						
Page Totals:						

VITAMINS/SUPPLEMENTS/MEDS.

Water: 1 2 3 4 5 6 7 8
(8 oz)

	Calories	Carbs (g)	Added Sugar (g)	Fiber (g)	Protein (g)	Fat (g)	
DINNER							
Time: Totals:							
SNACK							
Time: Totals:							
Grand Totals:							

PHYSICAL ACTIVITY

Activity	Duration	Intensity	Cal/Burn

BLOOD SUGAR LOG

	Before	After	Insulin
Breakfast			
Lunch			
Dinner			
Bedtime			

NOTES:

_____

_____

_____

_____

_____

Day: ☐   ____ / ____ / ____   Weight: ☐
                        (Date)

Sleep (hrs): 1 2 3 4 5 6 7 8

	Calories	Carbs (g)	Added Sugar (g)	Fiber (g)	Protein (g)	Fat (g)
BREAKFAST						
Time: Totals:						
SNACK						
Time: Totals:						
LUNCH						
Time: Totals:						
SNACK						
Time: Totals:						
Page Totals:						

VITAMINS/SUPPLEMENTS/MEDS.

Water: 1 2 3 4 5 6 7 8
(8 oz)

	Calories	Carbs (g)	Added Sugar (g)	Fiber (g)	Protein (g)	Fat (g)
DINNER						
Time: Totals:						
SNACK						
Time: Totals:						
Grand Totals:						

PHYSICAL ACTIVITY

Activity	Duration	Intensity	Cal/Burn

BLOOD SUGAR LOG

	Before	After	Insulin
Breakfast			
Lunch			
Dinner			
Bedtime			

NOTES:

Day: [ ] ____/____/____ Weight: [ ]

(Date)

Sleep (hrs): 1 2 3 4 5 6 7 8

	Calories	Carbs (g)	Added Sugar (g)	Fiber (g)	Protein (g)	Fat (g)
BREAKFAST						
Time: Totals:						
SNACK						
Time: Totals:						
LUNCH						
Time: Totals:						
SNACK						
Time: Totals:						
Page Totals:						

VITAMINS/SUPPLEMENTS/MEDS.

[ ]

Water: 1 2 3 4 5 6 7 8
(8 oz)

	Calories	Carbs (g)	Added Sugar (g)	Fiber (g)	Protein (g)	Fat (g)	
DINNER							
Time: Totals:							
SNACK							
Time: Totals:							
Grand Totals:							

PHYSICAL ACTIVITY

Activity	Duration	Intensity	Cal/Burn

BLOOD SUGAR LOG

	Before	After	Insulin
Breakfast			
Lunch			
Dinner			
Bedtime			

NOTES:

Day: [ ]   ____/____/____   Weight: [ ]

(Date)

Sleep (hrs): 1 2 3 4 5 6 7 8

	Calories	Carbs (g)	Added Sugar (g)	Fiber (g)	Protein (g)	Fat (g)
BREAKFAST						
Time: Totals:						
SNACK						
Time: Totals:						
LUNCH						
Time: Totals:						
SNACK						
Time: Totals:						
Page Totals:						

VITAMINS/SUPPLEMENTS/MEDS.

[ ]

Water: 1 2 3 4 5 6 7 8
(8 oz)

	Calories	Carbs (g)	Added Sugar (g)	Fiber (g)	Protein (g)	Fat (g)
DINNER						
Time: Totals:						
SNACK						
Time: Totals:						
Grand Totals:						

PHYSICAL ACTIVITY

Activity	Duration	Intensity	Cal/Burn

BLOOD SUGAR LOG

	Before	After	Insulin
Breakfast			
Lunch			
Dinner			
Bedtime			

NOTES:

Day: [ ]   ____ / ____ / ____   Weight: [ ]

(Date)

Sleep (hrs): 1 2 3 4 5 6 7 8

	Calories	Carbs (g)	Added Sugar (g)	Fiber (g)	Protein (g)	Fat (g)
BREAKFAST						
Time: Totals:						
SNACK						
Time: Totals:						
LUNCH						
Time: Totals:						
SNACK						
Time: Totals:						
Page Totals:						

VITAMINS/SUPPLEMENTS/MEDS.

Water: 1 2 3 4 5 6 7 8
(8 oz)

	Calories	Carbs (g)	Added Sugar (g)	Fiber (g)	Protein (g)	Fat (g)
DINNER						
Time: Totals:						
SNACK						
Time: Totals:						
Grand Totals:						

PHYSICAL ACTIVITY

Activity	Duration	Intensity	Cal/Burn

BLOOD SUGAR LOG

	Before	After	Insulin
Breakfast			
Lunch			
Dinner			
Bedtime			

NOTES:

_____
_____
_____
_____
_____

Day: [ ]   _____/_____/_____   Weight: [ ]

(Date)

Sleep (hrs): 1 2 3 4 5 6 7 8

	Calories	Carbs (g)	Added Sugar (g)	Fiber (g)	Protein (g)	Fat (g)
BREAKFAST						
Time: Totals:						
SNACK						
Time: Totals:						
LUNCH						
Time: Totals:						
SNACK						
Time: Totals:						
Page Totals:						

VITAMINS/SUPPLEMENTS/MEDS.

Water: 1 2 3 4 5 6 7 8
(8 oz)

DINNER	Calories	Carbs (g)	Added Sugar (g)	Fiber (g)	Protein (g)	Fat (g)	
Time: Totals:							
SNACK							
Time: Totals:							
Grand Totals:							

PHYSICAL ACTIVITY

Activity	Duration	Intensity	Cal/Burn

BLOOD SUGAR LOG

	Before	After	Insulin
Breakfast			
Lunch			
Dinner			
Bedtime			

NOTES:

Day: [ ]   ____/____/____   **Weight:** [ ]
(Date)

Sleep (hrs): 1 2 3 4 5 6 7 8

	Calories	Carbs (g)	Added Sugar (g)	Fiber (g)	Protein (g)	Fat (g)
BREAKFAST						
Time: Totals:						
SNACK						
Time: Totals:						
LUNCH						
Time: Totals:						
SNACK						
Time: Totals:						
Page Totals:						

VITAMINS/SUPPLEMENTS/MEDS.

Water: 1 2 3 4 5 6 7 8
(8 oz)

	Calories	Carbs (g)	Added Sugar (g)	Fiber (g)	Protein (g)	Fat (g)
DINNER						
Time: Totals:						
SNACK						
Time: Totals:						
Grand Totals:						

PHYSICAL ACTIVITY

Activity	Duration	Intensity	Cal/Burn

BLOOD SUGAR LOG

	Before	After	Insulin
Breakfast			
Lunch			
Dinner			
Bedtime			

NOTES:

Day: [ ]   ___/___/___   Weight: [ ]
(Date)

Sleep (hrs): 1 2 3 4 5 6 7 8

	Calories	Carbs (g)	Added Sugar (g)	Fiber (g)	Protein (g)	Fat (g)
BREAKFAST						
Time: Totals:						
SNACK						
Time: Totals:						
LUNCH						
Time: Totals:						
SNACK						
Time: Totals:						
Page Totals:						

VITAMINS/SUPPLEMENTS/MEDS.

Water: 1 2 3 4 5 6 7 8
(8 oz)

	Calories	Carbs (g)	Added Sugar (g)	Fiber (g)	Protein (g)	Fat (g)
DINNER						
Time: Totals:						
SNACK						
Time: Totals:						
Grand Totals:						

PHYSICAL ACTIVITY

Activity	Duration	Intensity	Cal/Burn

BLOOD SUGAR LOG

	Before	After	Insulin
Breakfast			
Lunch			
Dinner			
Bedtime			

NOTES:

Day: [ ]   ___/___/___   Weight: [   ]
                    (Date)

Sleep (hrs): 1 2 3 4 5 6 7 8

	Calories	Carbs (g)	Added Sugar (g)	Fiber (g)	Protein (g)	Fat (g)
BREAKFAST						
Time: Totals:						
SNACK						
Time: Totals:						
LUNCH						
Time: Totals:						
SNACK						
Time: Totals:						
Page Totals:						

VITAMINS/SUPPLEMENTS/MEDS.

Water: 1 2 3 4 5 6 7 8
(8 oz)

	Calories	Carbs (g)	Added Sugar (g)	Fiber (g)	Protein (g)	Fat (g)	
DINNER							
Time: Totals:							
SNACK							
Time: Totals:							
Grand Totals:							

PHYSICAL ACTIVITY

Activity	Duration	Intensity	Cal/Burn

BLOOD SUGAR LOG

	Before	After	Insulin
Breakfast			
Lunch			
Dinner			
Bedtime			

NOTES:

Day: [ ]   ____ / ____ / ____   Weight: [ ]

(Date)

Sleep (hrs): 1 2 3 4 5 6 7 8

	Calories	Carbs (g)	Added Sugar (g)	Fiber (g)	Protein (g)	Fat (g)
BREAKFAST						
Time: Totals:						
SNACK						
Time: Totals:						
LUNCH						
Time: Totals:						
SNACK						
Time: Totals:						
Page Totals:						

VITAMINS/SUPPLEMENTS/MEDS.

[ ]

Water: 1 2 3 4 5 6 7 8
(8 oz)

DINNER	Calories	Carbs (g)	Added Sugar (g)	Fiber (g)	Protein (g)	Fat (g)
Time: Totals:						
SNACK						
Time: Totals:						
Grand Totals:						

PHYSICAL ACTIVITY

Activity	Duration	Intensity	Cal/Burn

BLOOD SUGAR LOG

	Before	After	Insulin
Breakfast			
Lunch			
Dinner			
Bedtime			

NOTES:

Day: [ ] ____ / ____ / _____ Weight: [ ]

(Date)

Sleep (hrs): 1 2 3 4 5 6 7 8

	Calories	Carbs (g)	Added Sugar (g)	Fiber (g)	Protein (g)	Fat (g)
BREAKFAST						
Time: Totals:						
SNACK						
Time: Totals:						
LUNCH						
Time: Totals:						
SNACK						
Time: Totals:						
Page Totals:						

VITAMINS/SUPPLEMENTS/MEDS.

[ ]

Water: 1 2 3 4 5 6 7 8
(8 oz)

	Calories	Carbs (g)	Added Sugar (g)	Fiber (g)	Protein (g)	Fat (g)	
DINNER							
Time: Totals:							
SNACK							
Time: Totals:							
Grand Totals:							

PHYSICAL ACTIVITY

Activity	Duration	Intensity	Cal/Burn

BLOOD SUGAR LOG

	Before	After	Insulin
Breakfast			
Lunch			
Dinner			
Bedtime			

NOTES:

Day: [ ]   ____/____/____   **Weight:** [ ]

(Date)

Sleep (hrs): 1 2 3 4 5 6 7 8

	Calories	Carbs (g)	Added Sugar (g)	Fiber (g)	Protein (g)	Fat (g)
BREAKFAST						
Time: Totals:						
SNACK						
Time: Totals:						
LUNCH						
Time: Totals:						
SNACK						
Time: Totals:						
Page Totals:						

VITAMINS/SUPPLEMENTS/MEDS.

Water: 1 2 3 4 5 6 7 8
(8 oz)

	Calories	Carbs (g)	Added Sugar (g)	Fiber (g)	Protein (g)	Fat (g)
DINNER						
Time: Totals:						
SNACK						
Time: Totals:						
Grand Totals:						

PHYSICAL ACTIVITY

Activity	Duration	Intensity	Cal/Burn

BLOOD SUGAR LOG

	Before	After	Insulin
Breakfast			
Lunch			
Dinner			
Bedtime			

NOTES:

Day: [ ] ____/____/____ Weight: [ ]
(Date)

Sleep (hrs): 1 2 3 4 5 6 7 8

	Calories	Carbs (g)	Added Sugar (g)	Fiber (g)	Protein (g)	Fat (g)
BREAKFAST						
Time: Totals:						
SNACK						
Time: Totals:						
LUNCH						
Time: Totals:						
SNACK						
Time: Totals:						
Page Totals:						

VITAMINS/SUPPLEMENTS/MEDS.

Water: 1 2 3 4 5 6 7 8
(8 oz)

DINNER	Calories	Carbs (g)	Added Sugar (g)	Fiber (g)	Protein (g)	Fat (g)
Time: Totals:						
SNACK						
Time: Totals:						
Grand Totals:						

PHYSICAL ACTIVITY

Activity	Duration	Intensity	Cal/Burn

BLOOD SUGAR LOG

	Before	After	Insulin
Breakfast			
Lunch			
Dinner			
Bedtime			

NOTES:

Day: [ ]   ____/____/____   Weight: [ ]
                      (Date)

Sleep (hrs): 1 2 3 4 5 6 7 8

	Calories	Carbs (g)	Added Sugar (g)	Fiber (g)	Protein (g)	Fat (g)
BREAKFAST						
Time: Totals:						
SNACK						
Time: Totals:						
LUNCH						
Time: Totals:						
SNACK						
Time: Totals:						
Page Totals:						

VITAMINS/SUPPLEMENTS/MEDS.

Water: 1 2 3 4 5 6 7 8
(8 oz)

	Calories	Carbs (g)	Added Sugar (g)	Fiber (g)	Protein (g)	Fat (g)	
DINNER							
Time: Totals:							
SNACK							
Time: Totals:							
Grand Totals:							

PHYSICAL ACTIVITY

Activity	Duration	Intensity	Cal/Burn

BLOOD SUGAR LOG

	Before	After	Insulin
Breakfast			
Lunch			
Dinner			
Bedtime			

NOTES:

Day: ☐   ____/____/____   Weight: ☐
                    (Date)

Sleep (hrs): 1 2 3 4 5 6 7 8

	Calories	Carbs (g)	Added Sugar (g)	Fiber (g)	Protein (g)	Fat (g)	
BREAKFAST							
Time: Totals:							
SNACK							
Time: Totals:							
LUNCH							
Time: Totals:							
SNACK							
Time: Totals:							
Page Totals:							

VITAMINS/SUPPLEMENTS/MEDS.

Water: 1 2 3 4 5 6 7 8
(8 oz)

	Calories	Carbs (g)	Added Sugar (g)	Fiber (g)	Protein (g)	Fat (g)	
DINNER							
Time: Totals:							
SNACK							
Time: Totals:							
Grand Totals:							

PHYSICAL ACTIVITY

Activity	Duration	Intensity	Cal/Burn

BLOOD SUGAR LOG

	Before	After	Insulin
Breakfast			
Lunch			
Dinner			
Bedtime			

NOTES:

Day: [ ]   ____/____/____   Weight: [   ]
                      (Date)

Sleep (hrs): 1 2 3 4 5 6 7 8

	Calories	Carbs (g)	Added Sugar (g)	Fiber (g)	Protein (g)	Fat (g)
BREAKFAST						
Time: Totals:						
SNACK						
Time: Totals:						
LUNCH						
Time: Totals:						
SNACK						
Time: Totals:						
Page Totals:						

VITAMINS/SUPPLEMENTS/MEDS.

Water: 1 2 3 4 5 6 7 8
(8 oz)

	Calories	Carbs (g)	Added Sugar (g)	Fiber (g)	Protein (g)	Fat (g)	
DINNER							
Time: Totals:							
SNACK							
Time: Totals:							
Grand Totals:							

PHYSICAL ACTIVITY

Activity	Duration	Intensity	Cal/Burn

BLOOD SUGAR LOG

	Before	After	Insulin
Breakfast			
Lunch			
Dinner			
Bedtime			

NOTES:

Day: [ ]   ____/____/____   Weight: [ ]

(Date)

Sleep (hrs): 1 2 3 4 5 6 7 8

	Calories	Carbs (g)	Added Sugar (g)	Fiber (g)	Protein (g)	Fat (g)
BREAKFAST						
Time: Totals:						
SNACK						
Time: Totals:						
LUNCH						
Time: Totals:						
SNACK						
Time: Totals:						
Page Totals:						

VITAMINS/SUPPLEMENTS/MEDS.

Water: 1 2 3 4 5 6 7 8
(8 oz)

	Calories	Carbs (g)	Added Sugar (g)	Fiber (g)	Protein (g)	Fat (g)
DINNER						
Time: Totals:						
SNACK						
Time: Totals:						
Grand Totals:						

PHYSICAL ACTIVITY

Activity	Duration	Intensity	Cal/Burn

BLOOD SUGAR LOG

	Before	After	Insulin
Breakfast			
Lunch			
Dinner			
Bedtime			

NOTES:

Notes

Date: _____/_____/_____

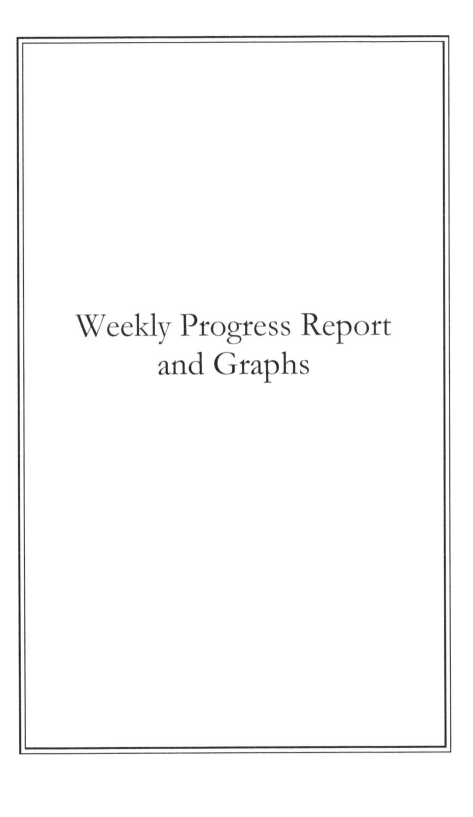

Weekly Progress Report
and Graphs

Weekly Progress Report and Graph

PROGRESS REPORT

Week	Date	Weight	Upper Arms	Chest	Waist	Hips	Thighs	
Week 1:								
Week 2:								
Week 3:								
Week 4:								
Week 5:								
Week 6:								
Week 7:								
Week 8:								
Week 9:								
Week 10:								
Week 11:								
Week 12:								
Week 13:								

Weight																
Week	1	2	3	4	5	6	7	8	9	10	11	12	13	14	15	16

Additional Graphs

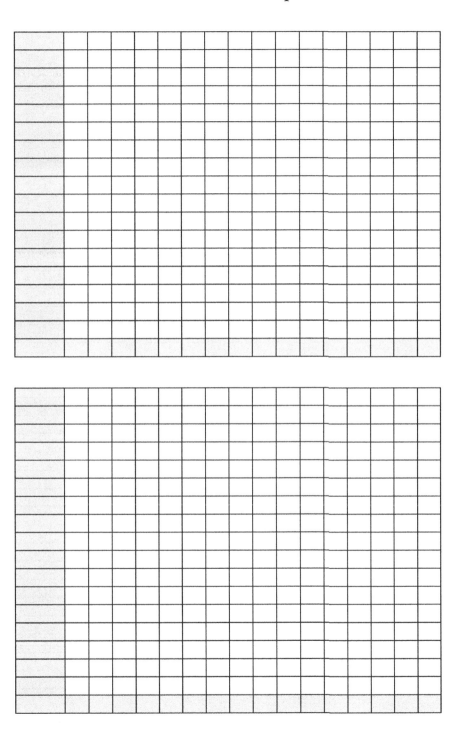

Notes

Date: _____/_____/_____

Nutrition Facts

NUTRITION FACTS

	Calories	Carbs (g)	Added Sugar (g)	Fiber (g)	Protein (g)	Fat (g)
FRUITS						
Apple, raw (1 medium, 2-3/4" across)	72	19	0	3	0	0
Apricots, raw (1 cup, halves)	74	17	0	3	0	0
Avocado, raw (1 cup)	240	13	0	10	3	0
Banana (1 medium, 7"-7-7/8" long)	105	27	0	3	1	0
Blueberries, raw (1 cup)	84	21	0	4	1	0
Cantaloupe, raw (1)	23	6	0	1	1	0
Cherries, sweet, raw (1 cup, with pits)	87	22	0	3	1	0
Grapefruit (1 medium - 4" across)	82	21	0	3	2	0
Grapes, raw, seedless (1 cup)	104	27	0	1	1	0
Honeydew melon, raw (1 cup)	61	15	0	1	1	0
Mango, raw (1 cup, sliced)	107	28	0	3	1	0
Nectarine, raw (1 cup, sliced)	63	15	0	2	2	0
Orange, raw (1 section or slice)	8	2	0	0	0	0
Papaya, raw (1 cup, cubes)	55	14	0	3	1	0
Peach, raw (1 cup)	66	16	0	3	2	0
Pear, raw (1 cup, sliced or cubed)	87	23	0	5	1	0
Pineapple, raw (1 cup, chunks)	82	22	0	2	1	0
Plum, raw (1 cup, sliced)	76	19	0	2	1	0
Prunes, dried, uncooked (1 cup)	418	111	0	12	4	0
Raisins (1 cup)	434	115	0	5	4	0
Raspberries, red, raw (1 cup)	64	15	0	8	1	0
Rasperries, black, raw (1 cup)	70	16	0	9	2	0
Strawberries (1 cup, whole)	46	11	0	3	1	0
Tangerine (1 cup, sections)	103	26	0	4	2	0
Watermelon, raw (1 cup, diced)	46	11	0	1	1	0
VEGETABLES						
Acorn squash, raw (1 cup)	56	15	0	2	1	0
Artichokes, stuffed (1 cup)	94	13	0	3	3	0
Asparagus, cooked, no salt/fat (1 cup)	40	7	0	4	4	0
Bean sprouts, cooked with salt (1 cup)	58	6	0	1	6	0

NUTRITION FACTS

VEGETABLES (CONT'D)	Calories	Carbs (g)	Added Sugar (g)	Fiber (g)	Protein (g)	Fat (g)
Brussel sprouts, cooked, no fat (1 cup)	56	11	0	4	4	0
Cabbage, cooked, no fat (1 cup)	35	8	0	3	2	0
Carrots, raw, chopped (1 cup)	52	12	0	4	1	0
Cauliflower, fresh, cooked, no fat (1 cup	33	6	0	3	3	0
Celery, raw (1 cup)	16	3	0	2	1	0
Collards, fresh, cooked, no fat (1 cup)	33	6	0	4	3	0
Corn, fresh, cooked, no fat (1 cup)	156	34	0	4	6	0
Cucumber, raw (1 cup)	14	3	0	1	1	0
Eggplant, cooked, no fat (1 cup)	34	8	0	2	1	0
Green beans, fresh, cooked, fat (1 cup)	44	10	0	4	2	0
Green lima beans, cooked, no fat (1 cup)	185	35	0	11	11	1
Green peas, cooked, no fat (1 cup)	133	25	0	9	9	0
Green peppers, raw (1 cup)	30	7	0	3	1	0
Iceberg lettuce, raw (1 cup)	8	2	0	1	0	0
Kale, fresh, cooked, no fat (1 cup)	36	7	0	3	2	1
Mushroom, cooked, no fat (1 cup)	44	8	0	3	3	1
Mustard greens, cooked, no fat (1 cup)	21	3	0	3	3	0
Okra, fresh, cooked, no fat (1 cup)	35	7	0	4	3	0
Onions, fresh, cooked, no fat (1 cup)	92	21	0	3	3	0
Potato, baked, peel eaten (1 cup)	112	26	0	1	3	0
Pumpkin, fresh, cooked (1 cup)	49	12	0	3	2	0
Red peppers, raw (1 cup)	46	9	0	3	1	0
Romain lettuce, raw (1 cup)	8	2	0	1	1	0
Spinach, raw (1 cup)	7	1	0	1	1	0
Squash, summer, cooked, no fat (1 cup)	36	8	0	3	2	1
Sweet potato, baked w/skin (1 medium)	226	52	0	9	5	0
Tomatoes, raw (1 cup)	22	5	0	1	1	0
Turnip greens, fresh, cooked, fat (1 cup)	29	6	0	5	2	0
Water chestnut (1 cup)	79	19	0	4	1	0
Watercress, cooked, no fat (1 cup)	15	2	0	1	3	0

NUTRITION FACTS

	Calories	Carbs(g)	Added Sugar (g)	Fiber (g)	Protein (g)	Fat (g)
WHOLE GRAINS						
Amaranth, flakes, cereal (1 cup)	134	27	0	4	6	3
Barley, cooked, no fat (1 cup)	198	46	0	6	4	1
Bread, 100% whole wheat (1 slice)	69	12	1	2	4	1
Buckwheat groats, cooked, no fat (1 cup)	155	33	0	5	6	1
Cornmeal, whole grain (1 cup)	442	94	0	9	10	4
Cracker, 100% whole wheat (1)	17	3	0	0	0	1
Millet, cooked, no fat (1 cup)	205	41	0	2	6	2
Oatmeal, regular, cooked, no fat (1 cup)	143	26	0	4	5	2
Pasta, whole wheat, tomato sauce (1 cup)	290	50	2	9	9	7
Popcorn, microwave, oil/butter (1 cup)	83	6	0	1	1	7
Quinoa, cooked (1 cup)	222	39	0	5	8	4
Rice, brown, regular, cooked, no fat (1 c)	215	44	0	4	5	2
Rice, wild, cooked, no fat (1 cup)	164	35	0	3	6	1
Rolls, 100% whole wheat (1 medium)	96	18	3	3	3	2
Tortilla, whole wheat (1 medium)	92	20	0	2	3	0
REFINED GRAINS						
Bread, pita (1 medium)	124	25	0	1	4	1
Bread, white (1 slice)	69	13	1	1	2	1
Couscous, plain, cooked, no fat (1 cup)	174	36	0	2	6	0
Grits, corn, regular, cooked no fat (1 cup)	109	24	0	1	2	1
Noodles, chow mein (1 cup)	237	26	0	2	4	14
Pretzel, hard, salted (1 oz)	106	22	0	1	3	1
Rice, white, regular, cooked, no fat (1 cup	204	44	0	1	4	0
Rolls, white, soft (1 medium)	100	18	2	1	3	2
Tortilla, corn (1 medium)	52	11	0	2	1	1

NUTRITION FACTS

	Calories	Carbs(g)	Added Sugar (g)	Fiber (g)	Protein (g)	Fat (g)
PROTEIN FOODS						
Lean cuts of meats (4 oz)						
Beef, steak, grilled/broiled	208	0	0	0	34	7
Ham, fresh, cooked	238	0	0	0	33	11
Lamb, roast, cooked (4 oz)	223	0	0	0	30	10
Pork, chop, broiled/baked/grilled	222	0	0	0	31	10
Veal, roasted	197	0	0	0	30	8
Poultry (4 oz)						
Chicken, breast, no bone/skin, baked	184	0	0	0	34	4
Chicken, breast, no bone/skin, fried	215	0	0	0	35	8
Chicken, leg quarter, baked with skin	261	0	0	0	29	15
Duck, cooked., skin eaten	381	0	0	0	21	32
Turkey, white meat, roasted, no skin	222	0	0	0	32	9
Beans and Peas (cooked from dry)						
Black beans, no fat (1 cup)	198	36	0	9	12	1
Black-eye peas, no fat (1 cup)	158	33	0	8	5	1
Chickpeas, no fat (1 cup)	295	49	0	14	16	5
Kidney beans, no fat (1 cup)	217	39	0	13	15	1
Lentils, cooked, no fat (1 cup)	220	38	0	15	17	1
Lima beans, no fat (1 cup)	210	38	0	13	14	1
Pinto beans, no fat (1 cup)	199	36	0	9	12	1
Soybeans, no fat (1 cup)	310	18	0	11	30	16
Split peas, no fat (1 cup)	229	41	0	16	16	1
White beans, no fat (1 cup)	242	44	0	11	17	1
Processed Soy Products						
Tofu, breaded, fried (1 slice)	44	3	0	0	2	3
Veggie (soy) burger, no bun (1 patty)	124	10	0	3	11	4
Tempeh, raw (1 oz)	55	3	0	1	5	3
Texturized vegetable protein, dry (1 cup)	224	26	0	12	32	1
Nuts and Seeds						
Almonds, dry roasted (1 oz)	169	5	0	3	6	15
Cashews, roasted (1 oz)	165	9	0	1	5	14

NUTRITION FACTS

PROTEIN FOODS (CONT'D)	Calories	Carbs(g)	Added Sugar (g)	Fiber (g)	Protein (g)	Fat (g)
Nuts and Seeds (Cont'd)						
Hazelnuts (1 portion - 10 nuts)	88	2	0	1	2	9
Mixed nuts, dry roasted (1 cup)	814	35	0	12	24	70
Peanut butter (1 tbsp)	94	3	0	1	4	8
Peanuts, dry roasted (1 cup)	854	31	0	12	35	73
Pecans (1 oz)	196	4	0	3	3	20
Pistachios (1 oz)	160	8	0	3	6	13
Pumpkin seeds, roasted (1 tbsp)	81	2	0	1	4	7
Sesame seeds (tbsp)	53	2	0	2	2	5
Sunflower seeds, dry roasted, hulled (1 tbsp)	47	2	0	1	2	4
Walnuts (1 oz)	185	4	0	2	4	18
Seafood						
Catfish, battered, fried (4 oz)	275	8	0	0	17	19
Cod, battered, fried (4 oz)	196	8	0	0	20	9
Flounder, baked/broiled with oil (4 oz)	157	0	0	0	25	6
Haddock, baked/broiled, no fat (4 oz)	120	0	0	0	26	1
Herring, baked/broiled, no fat (4 oz)	222	0	0	0	25	13
Mackerel, baked/broiled, no fat (4 oz)	259	0	0	0	26	16
Porgy, baked/broiled, no fat (4 oz)	148	0	0	0	26	4
Salmon, baked/broiled, no fat (4 oz)	166	0	0	0	28	5
Sea bass, baked/broiled, no fat (4 oz)	139	0	0	0	26	3
Swordfish, baked/broiled, no fat (4 oz)	173	0	0	0	28	6
Trout, baked/broiled, no fat (4 oz)	189	0	0	0	28	7
Tuna, fresh, baked/broiled, no fat (4 oz)	148	0	0	0	32	1
Shellfish						
Clams, boiled/steamed (1 cup/12 medium)	138	5	0	0	24	2
Crab, steamed (1 cup - flaked)	119	0	0	0	24	2
Crayfish, boiled/steamed (1 cup)	113	0	0	0	23	2

NUTRITION FACTS

	Calories	Carbs(g)	Added Sugar (g)	Fiber (g)	Protein (g)	Fat (g)	
PROTEIN FOODS (CONT'D)							
Shellfish (Cont'd)							
Lobster, steamed/boiled (1 medium/2.5 lb)	286	4	0	0	60	2	
Mussels, steamed/poached (1 cup)	257	11	0	0	35	7	
Octopus, steamed (4 oz)	185	5	0	0	34	2	
Oyster, Eastern, steamed (1)	10	1	0	0	1	0	
Scallop, baked/broiled/grilled no fat (1)	14	0	0	0	3	0	
Squid, steamed/boiled (1 cup)	147	5	0	0	25	2	
Shrimp, steamed/boiled (1 cup)	200	2	0	0	38	3	
DAIRY							
Milk							
Fat-free, skim (1 cup)	83	12	0	0	8	0	
Low fat, 1% (4 oz)	102	12	0	0	8	2	
Reduced fat, 2% (1 cup)	122	12	0	0	8	5	
Whole milk (1 cup)	149	12	0	0	8	8	
Soy (1 cup)	108	12	0	0	6	4	
Cheese							
Cheddar cheese (1 oz)	114	0	0	0	7	9	
Mozzarella, low sodium (1 oz)	79	1	0	0	8	5	
Swiss (1 oz)	108	2	0	0	8	8	
Parmesan, hard (1 oz)	111	1	0	0	10	7	
Ricotta, part skim (1 oz)	39	1	0	0	3	2	
Cottage cheese, low fat, 1-2% (1 oz)	20	1	0	0	4	0	
American processed cheese	94	2	0	0	5	7	
Yogurt							
Fat-free, plain (8 oz)	127	17	0	0	13	0	
Low fat, plain (8 oz)	143	16	0	0	12	4	
Whole milk, plain (8 oz)	138	11	0	0	8	7	

NUTRITION FACTS

	Calories	Carbs (g)	Added Sugar (g)	Fiber (g)	Protein (g)	Fat (g)
COMMONLY EATEN FOODS						

Thank you for choosing

Food Journal & Blood Sugar Log

by I. S. Anderson

Other Titles by I. S. Anderson

Change Your Life Guided Journal

Food & Fitness Journal

**Health Journal: Discover Food Intolerances
and Allergies**

Workout Journal: Interval Training

Password Log

For inquiries or to provide feedback, contact:
nahjpress@outlook.com

Made in the USA
Monee, IL
15 December 2020